AF609313

Cancer InsideOut

Cancer InsideOut

An Insider's View of Chemo & Outsider's Guide for Support

Linda Crill

Opus INTL Media
Chico, CA

Published by
Opus INTL Media
www.CancerInsideOut.com

Library of Congress Cataloging-in-Publication Data
Crill, Linda
Cancer InsideOut: An Insider's View of Chemo & Outsider's Guide for Support/
Linda Crill.

Library of Congress Control Number 2025920333

ISBN 978-0-9858985-4-0 (hardcover)
ISBN 978-0-9858985-6-4 (paperback)
ISBN 978-0-9858985-5-7 (eBook)

Printed in the United States of America

To everyone who makes life a little easier for people with cancer, one caring act at a time.

Contents

Preface

WE ALL HAVE FEARS we hope we'll never face. For most, cancer is one of those. When we hear that someone we know or love is facing cancer and especially its difficult treatment chemotherapy, we want to contribute in some way to make their journey easier.

But how do we support others when we don't know what these experiences are really like? And, how do we approach them, when we don't know what to say, or worse, are afraid we'll say or do the wrong thing?

I've had cancer three times. I've gone through radiation, chemotherapy, and multiple surgeries. I've been the caregiver for a husband with terminal cancer. I speak to groups about the personal side of cancer. One of the most frequently asked questions by audiences is a variation of, "How can I help others who are experiencing cancer?"

Going through chemotherapy infusions in a new city with few local friends or support groups, I needed a way to express what I was experiencing during my 15 weeks of infusion chemotherapy. My chemo journal became the friend I told my innermost thoughts.

Later, when I shared some of these journal entries, I was surprised by the responses. Even people who had helped their spouse or family during chemotherapy said, "Your description of the treatments are familiar, but I never knew what was going on inside of my loved one."

The first part of this book, "An Insider's View," is a collection of select journal entries that share my own journey through chemotherapy. They tell about the hardships but also provide insight into some of the lighthearted moments while one is experiencing these treatments.

The second part, "Cancer Etiquette," is about what to say and not say to a person with cancer. Etiquette guidelines have been written to help us understand how to appropriately act in a variety of social situations. So why not use suggested cancer etiquette to help us understand how to behave and communicate with a person experiencing cancer and its challenging treatments?

Finally, the third part, "Supporting Others," is a list of 50+ ways to support those going through cancer and its treatments. We often give the blanket offer of: "Let me know what I can do to support you." Or, we show up with an unsolicited meal. But for someone going through extended treatments with health limitations, there are dozens of additional ways to help make their journey better.

This book presents both an insider's view of a cancer patient's internal journey through chemotherapy and treatments, and an outsider's guide to supporting a family member, friend, or someone you've heard about that is undergoing cancer care.

PART 1:
An Insider's View

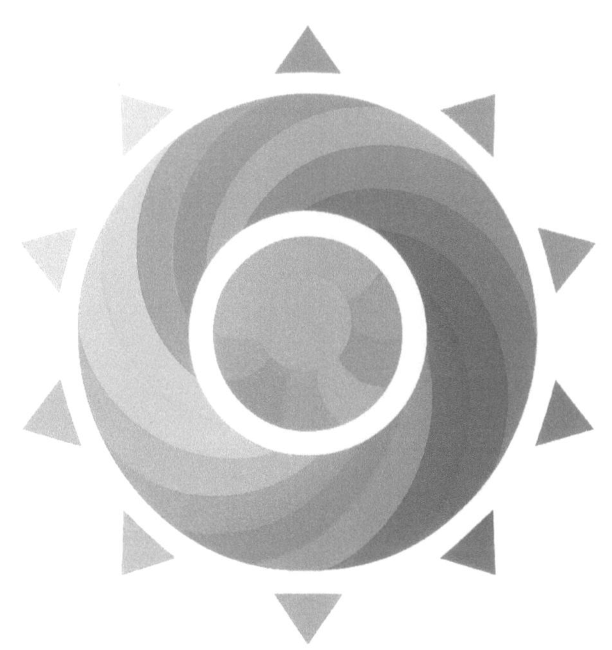

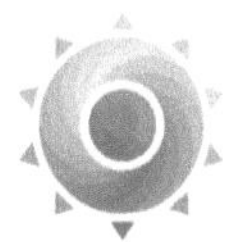

Hello Journal

March 1

CHEMOTHERAPY IS CHANGING my life. Before starting infusion treatments on February 15, doing anything active was always more attractive than sitting quietly and searching for words to write about what I was experiencing. Now, during the daytime, I can hardly find a reason to leave my chair.

Too tired to read someone else's words, the pile of unread books on my side table grows taller with each additional week of chemotherapy.

Too concerned about my compromised immune system, I've quit going to indoor group activities.

Too new in town to have deep enough friendships for them to insist on dropping by or reaching out to engage me in their activities. I look at my phone, but don't call anyone. *I don't want to be a bother.*

But if I don't have conversation, I need another way to explore my feelings and express myself. I pick up a new journal sporting cheerful flowers on its hardback cover. Inside are blank pages that beckon, "Fill me." However, I feel unable to even begin and consider regifting it to another who could.

Inside such a beautiful, formal book, I feel its entries need to be special, memorable, inspirational, and most of all well written. But my words are just a jumble of disjointed feelings and thoughts. Nothing that's neatly phrased, particularly brilliant or enlightening.

Still, it's my only companion today, so I pick up a pen and with my palm crease open her curved, lifted, empty pages. I feel deep inside myself and search for parts of me that need a voice.

Most of my entries aren't neat. My handwriting changes from one paragraph to the next, making them look as if they've been written by different people. There are unfinished sentences left hanging. Cross outs pepper entries like the splatter paintings I created as a child. I can't even crumple up false starts and toss them like I do with loose paper because her pages are firmly sewn into the spine.

But collectively, this book and the writings it holds, have become my best friend. She always listens to whatever I say and never interrupts or corrects me with thoughts of her own. My journal simply mirrors back to me the many inner voices translated into written words so I can remember, reread, and dive even deeper.

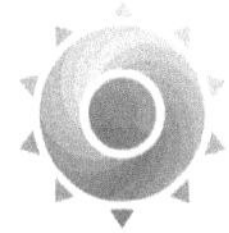

Blocked Expression

March 2

I'VE NEVER WRITTEN poetry. But now the feelings inside me are so intense that my normal writing feels too regimented. The following is the first entry I wrote in my journal. Each line flowed quickly from my pen, written as I felt it. When I stopped to observe the page, I was shocked to see what looked like a poem. My first one ever.

So many feelings
without words to express.

I feel the growing knot in my throat
where they stop and back up.

I want to hear
what they have to say.

But words don't come,
feelings don't express,
here I sit blocked.

I pick up my pen and say,
tell me what's there

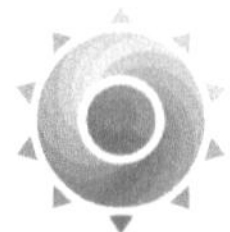

The Gravity of My Chair

March 8

MY PROBLEM IS OVERCOMING the heaviness of wanting to do nothing more than rest in my chair, cuddled up in blankets, and let the TV, Facebook, or staring out the window marginally entertain me.

I feel best about myself when I accomplish something. It can be as simple as exercising, cleaning, walking, or learning anything new.

The price I pay when my body isn't forced into activity, it becomes even more lethargic and heavy.

A headache grows.

Restlessness and boredom set in.

Any simple movement out of my chair opens a happier world.

But here I sit cemented in it, searching for that super energy to pull me free of its powerful gravity.

A minor victory is my hand reaches down to the remote and clicks off the TV.

I marvel at its independence and intelligence.

Now to the kitchen to make the soup that I've had the ingredients waiting for weeks, or to the office to tackle one of my to-do lists with no checked off items.

I throw out my imaginary climbing rope in the direction of the kitchen to pull my body free of my chair's powerful gravity.

I need to do more today than just sit.

From Superwoman to Just Plain Ordinary

March 12

WHEN I AGREED TO START the chemotherapy infusion treatments on February 28, of this year, I told myself, I don't have to experience the common chemo side effects of this journey that everyone complains about. After all, I'm an athlete, a meditator, used to previous difficult cancer treatments, and most of all, I've always healed faster than others by using my positive can-do mindset.

My friends and family send me encouraging messages that repeat variations of the phrases: "You can do this. You're not like others. You're strong!"

This morning, 34 days into my 84-day chemotherapy infusion treatments, I don't feel strong. I feel damn ordinary.

My head aches after a night of continually interrupted sleep. This morning's Tylenol and coffee don't offer their expected relief. Thanks to chemo my tongue is swollen and taste is gone except for an intense desire for sweets and salt. My nose bleeds at the slightest provocation. And exhaustion is the shadow I never shake.

I no longer feel like a superwoman able to leap over obstacles that block all others. I can't be the role model for rising above adversity that defeats most people.

This morning my symptoms, reactions, and exhaustion are classic—shared by my peers who face this same solution for eliminating cancer.

It's disappointing to be ordinary. And, it's a relief to accept what I'm experiencing without the need to overcome, rise above, or defeat it!

This is not a *battle* against cancer.

A *fight* to be won.

I'm not a *warrior* woman engaged in a *war*.

This is merely a journey of putting one foot in front of the other and checking off one more day on the treatment calendar as I trudge toward my last day of chemotherapy.

Today, it's finally time to be just ordinary, surrounded by my peers and those who came before us creating this well-worn footpath. We follow their footsteps with respect and gratitude for the improvements learned from their experiences, to make ours better and future treatments even more effective.

My infusion journey at least has a final date of completion. For many of my fellow walkers on this same path, their steps may be cut short by an ended life or extended into perpetuity in the hope they'll live just a little bit longer.

I have much to be grateful for and have great compassion for my fellow travelers—many carrying even heavier backpacks than my own. Next to them I walk in awe and cheer on all others.

I have said that this chemo was going to be a spiritual journey. But I'm discovering that this is a wider healing experience for me than just surviving this chemo treatment and cancer.

My heart is opening toward others. My old, outdated ways are crumbling. And now, it's time to just feel RAW.

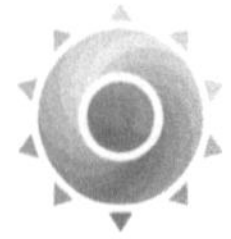

Wig Buying

March 13

ODDLY, MY GREATEST FEAR about needing infusion chemotherapy wasn't the chemo. I mourned the potential loss of my long blonde-silver hair that now flows down to the middle of my back. One thing I like about its length is the many ways to style it. Up in a swinging ponytail that pokes out the back of my sun hat, swept back from my face and held on the sides with colorful combs, or simply flowing long and free.

Last week at my second of four chemo treatments scheduled three weeks apart, I learned that now I can expect my hair to shed heavily. Already when I brush my hair, I hold a fist full of hair in my hand afterward.

The date of my new local friends' wedding is three weeks from today. And since it's outdoors, it will be safer and more possible for me to attend with my compromised immune system. Since I'm new in Chico, California, this will be a great opportunity to meet new people. Most of all, I want to make a good impression, be approachable, and not be remembered as the balding woman going through cancer.

I already have my dress, shoes, and jewelry picked out. I even decided to buy the right dark green polish for my nails. More than anything, I want to go to this wedding looking normal. But what about my head? No part of my outfit planning included wearing a cancer cap to hide my baldness. And stylish hats always have a person's hair showing beneath it somewhere. I'll have little to none by then.

It's obviously time to start to think about buying a wig so I'll have it when I need it next month and beyond.

I've researched wigs online to get an idea of what's available, costs, and types. There are many websites and a profusion of styles, colors, shapes, and cuts. Having bought clothing online, I know that the way a garment looks on a model in a photo can be shockingly dissimilar to what arrives in the mail, and how it looks on me. Fit, color, and quality can be disappointing.

I know I will not be an easy person to please. I've noticed so many ill-fitting wigs over my lifetime and always said to myself, *I'd never do that!* But I'm forced to erase another "never-do-that statement" from my beliefs. I tell myself: *One necessary condition of any wig I buy is, it must look as if it is really my hair.*

My sister Anita and I head to the local wig shop confident that this is the better approach. On our arrival, a salesperson tries to help by giving me different styles to try on. What I hadn't considered is how sensitive my head has become to any touch. Pulling on tight, ill-fitting, one-size-fits-all wigs is not only physically painful but emotionally upsetting. Most are in dark colors and look nothing like my light-colored hair. All clearly look like wigs and feel brittle and synthetic—totally unlike my natural hair.

In the Central Valley of Northern California, our summer weeks can easily reach the high 90s and sometimes even over 110 degrees. These synthetic hair wigs are like wearing a heavy, wool stocking cap that doesn't breathe and holds in my body heat. I can't imagine what it would be like to wear one of these in the summer.

We leave our local wig shop without buying anything. I am determined to go to a bigger city where I can try on natural hair wigs with a ventilated cap holding its hair.

I am grateful that I still have time to shop again for a better choice.

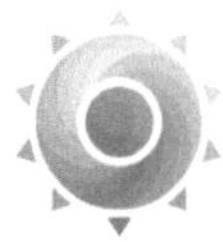

Gratitude–Opposite Perspectives

March 14

SITTING IN MY CHAIR, I WATCH as the colors of trees and sky fade and begin to soften gently in the scene outside my window. Dusk is my favorite time of day. Tonight, the sky has a pink glow that imbues and repaints the colorings of everything below it.

I feel my heart opening and resting after a difficult day of recuperation following my second chemotherapy infusion just five days ago. My sister Anita left this morning to drive 11 hours back to her home in the high desert in Southern California.

This is the third time she has driven 600 miles each way to support me during this cancer journey. As a sister and hospice nurse for over 20 years, she insisted on being with me during my mastectomy last December. Now she has been at my first and second chemotherapy infusions. And with both infusions she stayed another five days to help me through the difficult post-infusion days filled with ever-changing reactions.

It starts with just one thought, *I'm grateful for my sister Anita.* As I sit thinking about her selfless support, this initial feeling of gratitude builds and extends to her husband Bruce, who encouraged her to come and be with me while he stayed at home and meditated for my healing and returned health.

Next, I look at the pink, mini, six-inch-long boxing gloves hanging on the ladder, leaning against my front room wall, that holds a collection of four lap blankets. These were dropped off by Dee, a new friend from Newcomers Club, after she heard I couldn't attend their large indoor monthly luncheon meetings due to my compromised immune system.

Suddenly, I feel like the person at the Emmy Awards wanting to thank everyone who helped them along the way. My overwhelming feelings of gratitude keep encompassing more circumstances and people.

My neighbor, Sandy, who when she heard my hands were cold and I wished I had a pair of gloves with no fingers, four hours later, brought me a pair she had spent the previous hours knitting.

My oncologist, Dr. Nicole Whitlatch, who has always given me more time than the standard 15-minute doctor visit. And when I commented about how hard her job must be to continuously deliver difficult news, her response was, "It's a privilege to serve." Wow! That's not the response I was expecting.

And the Enloe cancer nurses and office workers who call me back, often after 6:30 pm, to answer a question I left on their voice mail earlier that day. They apologize for calling me so late.

When I say, "Didn't your office close at 4:00 pm? Why are you still working so late?"

They reply, "It's important to get back to you, and this was the first time all day that I could."

Then there is the American Cancer Society who gave me hotel vouchers for doctor visits over three hours away by car so that I wouldn't have to drive for six hours in addition to sitting through a long appointment, all in one day. They also paid for my sister Anita to stay in a hotel during my cancer surgery.

My hiking, pickleball, and kayak buddies who, when it gets too hot and I take off my hat, treat me normally at the sight of my balding head. One time walking back to the car after a too aggressive (for me) hike, I hooked my arm into my hiking friend Laura's arm and ended up holding her hand until we reached my car. I needed that extra support, she gave it and understood without my asking.

And Medicare and my Med Supp insurance. I never thought I'd praise the government or insurance companies, but I never could have paid all of these medical bills without them. I don't see the bills unless I log onto their sites. But I know this cancer journey has cost in the millions, and it's paid for except for the few extra prescriptions I need to fill at the local pharmacy.

As I write this more and more ideas keep gathering inside me. I started with a single feeling of great thankfulness for my sister's sacrifices. But now so many others explode in my mind. I'm even grateful for the socks on my feet—those funny green avocados on a deep purple background just make me smile. And socks make me think of my younger daughter Lindsey who loves funny socks. I'm grateful for her flying out from Washington, D.C. to California to be with me for several weeks post-surgery. And of course, Lindsey makes me think of my other two daughters, Kim and Heather, whose FaceTime calls and hats to cover my balding head have meant so much. Then there are the family emails from my other sister Carol and FaceTime calls and messages from my Venezuelan family and close friends.

Help! Where do I stop? I'm glowing inside and radiating love. My constant headache dissolves in the wake of this overwhelming feeling of gratitude. I feel privileged to be honored by so much support.

This morning, as I write in this journal, I realize something else, something very special. This gratitude is what I needed to silence the "why me?" Or even stronger, the "why me for the third time?" I know well how these questions can take me quickly down a slide to self-pity and anger.

A year ago, I was invited to a new friend's home for dinner. One of the other dinner guests was a minister at a local church. She excitedly talked about the gratitude walk she had helped to organize and lead that afternoon at our local public park.

They had arranged for multiple stations where walkers stopped to perform assignments led by volunteer facilitators. At the stop where she was in charge, people stood on a small bridge and were instructed to release all negative thoughts and feelings into the flowing stream below. Then they were told to breathe in gratitude and happiness before walking to the next station.

I remember thinking, *Yep, I'm really in California.* I was pleased by how much the event had meant to her and my fellow dinner companions, but I was secretly relieved that I hadn't participated. I couldn't imagine needing to attend a group event to accomplish this.

At our local OLLI university program for seniors, there is a four-session course on gratitude. I had heard past participants raving about this class. But I skipped it and chose from other areas of interest. Again, it simply seemed unnecessary to me.

Please, I don't want to be a Grinch of Thanks-giving traditions with everyone being asked to say what they're grateful for before eating a huge meal. I've forced my family and guests to do this on more than one year in the past.

Daily, and often before falling asleep at night, I look for the things to be grateful for and give thanks for them. But the thought of forcing a focus on gratitude in a class or group walk was outside my comfort zone.

That's the problem with any tools or methods to help people soothe and alleviate some of the challenges faced in life. In one situation they feel superfluous and unnecessary. And in the next, they become lifelines for getting through one more day of a difficult journey.

This is one of the paradoxes of writing in this journal. I started out needing to express gratitude for my sister, and now I've wandered through many more paragraphs with ever expanding views. Whoever thinks writing is a lonely activity doesn't have my brain. It can argue and even disagree with itself.

I close this journal entry circling back to my opening observations about how many wonderful gifts are being given to me on this journey. Gifts that I never asked for. I'm truly blessed.

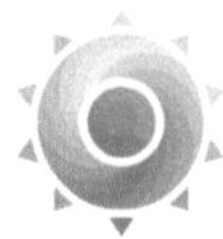

It's Easy to Lose the Whole Me

March 20

THE FIRST THING I DO, as I awaken and slowly emerge from my dream world, is recognize whether I'm still alive on this earth and not in some other alternate reality. As I become more fully conscious and remember my current chemo journey, I ask: *Am I okay? Today will I have new or deteriorating symptoms to deal with as my body continues its decline from more days of treatments?*

I scan my body starting at my head and progressing toward my feet, stopping at yesterday's trouble spots to give them special attention. My nose for bleeding or my throat for its thick coating. I also pause any place that feels even a tiny bit different to ascertain whether it's a new concern or merely my imagination.

At breakfast, this focus on my body persists as I try to eat with a tongue that is raw, swollen, and dislikes any non-soft texture or too-hot temperature.

Sitting in my chair after eating I think, *Oh, yeah! How are my emotions and mind when I'm not focused solely on my physical body? Didn't I used to have other morning feelings, like excitement for the day ahead or ideas about activities I had planned?*

But now, I simply focus on the headache between my eyebrows, wondering how to dissolve it. Mechanically, I reach up and begin rubbing in small circles. Headaches are so common. I've given up wondering why they occur, and I never focus on them for long. Instead, I encourage any other new ideas to surface and distract me.

I dream of a time when I will no longer think about my health and body 24/7. When the day's activities aren't dominated by endless medical appointments, support groups, lab tests, and taking medications—then dealing with their side effects. A time when talking and texting with family and friends doesn't begin with them wanting honest answers to "How are you?" A time when my physical body fades to the background and allows a spotlight to shine on other areas of my life. *After all, more parts of my life still exist somewhere. Don't they?*

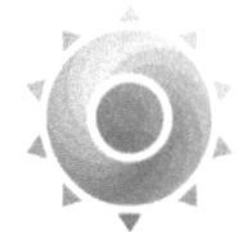

Ain't Gonna Study War No More

March 21

I GREW UP IN A FAMILY and church that loved to sing. It could be a way of passing time on long family drives, sitting around a campfire when camping, or sharing fellowship together at a church potluck supper or summer picnic.

We children especially enjoyed singing along with adults when the songs were easy to remember, funny, or sung loudly with enthusiasm.

One song that popped into my head this morning from my long ago past is "Ain't Gonna Study War No More."

> I'm gonna lay down my sword and shield
> Down by the riverside (3x)
> I'm gonna lay down my sword and shield
> Down by the riverside, study war no more.

Chorus
I ain't gonna study war no more
Ain't gonna study war no more (2x)
I ain't gonna study war no more
Ain't gonna study war no more (2x)

This song was always sung by everyone with great jubilation and especially by the generation that had just gone through WWII. Their fervor was so strong that we kids quickly got caught up in their energies.

But why are these words and its tune playing in my head this morning? I smile. It is because I've quit fighting the war against my cancer.

No, I'm not surrendering to cancer. I still want to rid my body of these errant cells. But viewing cancer as an *enemy to fight* and living daily on its *battlefield battling* this scary enemy takes precious energy I need for healing, living, and making it through each day.

Energy is the gold I miserly protect these days. It leaks out of me with every physical, mental, and emotional activity I engage in—both good and bad. When I'm in a tense, constantly-fighting negative state, I use up more energy than when I'm in a more relaxed, mellow, positive one.

When I was diagnosed with cancer the first time, 12 years ago, the tumor was only the size of a pea. The lab test said its rate of cellular division was less than 5%. Less than 10% is considered great because that means the cancer is growing extremely slowly.

My doctor teasingly said, "It's growing so slowly that we could even wait six months before removing it."

After a long pause while he processed my panicked look, he then quickly added, "But we're not going to do that."

Like most of us when we're diagnosed with cancer, I wanted these dangerous invading cells out of my body immediately. I was ready to march onto the *battlefield* and go to *war* against them. If the surgery for their removal could have been scheduled for that afternoon, I would have said, "Do it!"

With each of my three cancer surgeries, there was a relief after each surgery when the surgeons said, "We got it."

This chemo is to search out rogue cancer cells that may have metastasized (or in simple layperson's English, moved from my breast to another area of my body through the blood system).

In 1971, President Nixon proclaimed a *war* on cancer and signed the National Cancer Act. He used the term *war* because he equated cancer to be a national priority similar to any war effort.

This popular *war* vernacular has been further popularized by organizations raising money for cancer research and support for people with cancer. We, the people with cancer, are engaged in a *war* against our cancer. We *fight* a *battle* against our cancer that needs to be won at all costs. We're *soldiers, warriors, militants* engaged in constant *combat.*

These powerful words incite the adrenalin in my body as I gear up 24/7 for a tough fight against this predatory enemy inside my own body. It fuels my anger against these invading cancerous cells that I visualize as enemies trying to take over and crowd out healthy ones.

With this constantly churning combat and war mindset fueled by anger and fear, it's difficult to slow down my racing thoughts, relax my tight muscles, and let myself rest peacefully. It's hard not to wake up multiple times each night thinking about cancer. I often sleep fitfully and have bad dreams. It feels as though I'm developing PTSD.

Finally, I pound my fist on my chair's arm and shout, "Enough of this war mentality! I ain't gonna study war no more, no more!"

Whew! I let out a huge sigh and along with it shed my fighting guns, heavy armor, and ammunition. Retreating, I leave this battle and head AWOL for home.

How can I heal if my precious energy is being spent in and drained by the wrong mindset and actions? To heal, my ammunition is no longer going to be fear and anger. Now it's going to be love, peace, and confidence in my strong body.

I shut my eyes and imagine white light pouring down over my body caressing it and filling every cell. I begin conversations with it that sound like a cooing mother soothing her small child who has awakened from a bad dream in the middle of the night.

I hug myself and repeat, "You're such a strong, wonderful body. Look at all we've been through together. I know you're dealing with a lot with this treatment. But I love you, and I'm going to be here with you caring for you as we experience chemo and healing together."

I stop multiple times during the day to talk to my body and praise it for its strengths. I envision and send loving energy to all areas of my body.

Something interesting is happening with my changed mindset. I'm no longer angry at the cancer cells. They're a part of me, too. They're merely cells with broken programming.

In the chemotherapy literature I received describing the two different types of medicine that are infused into my body, it explained that inside each cell is a mechanism that senses whether there are cells surrounding it. When it notices a gap around its cell, it divides. In my cancer cells, this mechanism is broken, and that's why some of my cells keep dividing when it's not needed. And of course, when a broken cancer cell divides, the resulting new ones carry this same malfunction.

So, I tell my cancer cells that they're damaged and that they're not needed. I visualize my immune system identifying them and removing them the same way it removes other old, tired cells and any with false programming. I envision the chemo fluids in my body supporting this elimination as well.

Praising and supporting my body, I'm more relaxed. I'm happier again instead of tense and fighting. My view of the world around me is more peaceful, too.

A major focus in my life is healing, and I believe this healthy, positive approach to daily living will fuel my body with energy to cure my body of cancer.

I download the song to my phone so I can remember the additional verses to this song. I vaguely remember a Nat King Cole version in the 1950s which he sang like a spiritual. I also remember Pete Seeger's anti-war version in the 1960s. But when not listening to these downloaded versions, I'm singing the version I sang with my family, fellow campers, and church members, “I ain’t going to study war no more.”

This is how I choose to heal and be healthy in mind, body, and spirit.

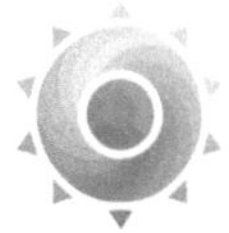

What's the Best Alternative—Sit or Explore?

March 22

IN LIFE, WHEN MAKING DECISIONS the choices aren't always between the good and bad ones. Sometimes all the alternatives appear undesirable.

At the beginning of February, before I learned I would need to go through chemotherapy, I thought I was through with cancer—having survived cancer surgery in December and its eight weeks of recovery ending in February. I excitedly signed up for a hiking class for women. The first class would be a classroom orientation followed by six different weekly 4- to 7-mile hikes.

I signed up to hopefully meet more local people, make new hiking friends, and learn where to go to explore and hike in the mountains and valleys around my new home in Northern California.

Instead of having cancer behind me post-surgery, I learned that I would need 15 weeks of chemo. I considered canceling my hiking class enrollment. Then I thought, *why not wait and see before each hike if I had the energy to do it?*

Today is the first day of class—the orientation session. In an email sent before the first session, we were instructed to come to class dressed as if we were going on a day-hike, and to bring our backpack filled with the usual gear we'd take on a hike.

This morning, I sat at home in my comfortable chair trying to tune in on my body and asked, *What do you need?* It begged me to continue sitting all day and miss my 1:00-3:30 hiking orientation class.

Even though my body kept signaling me that it wanted rest, it refused to sleep. I became bored after a morning of inactivity and knew the tedium would only grow worse if I stayed all afternoon in my chair. *Do I stay bored or force myself to go to class where I'll probably be miserable because I'll be too tired?* Neither option felt like a good one.

Frustrated and caught between two bad choices, I forced myself to change into hiking clothes, packed my backpack, and drove to my class, while reminding myself, *I can leave early if I need to.*

When we introduced ourselves, I shared that I was going through chemotherapy and didn't know if I would be able to hike very well as the treatments advanced.

As I listened in class and participated for an hour, my body began begging me for sleep, but I ignored its seduction and stayed awake.

At the end of the session, several participants and the two leaders came over to me to say they were glad I had decided to stay enrolled.

Now that today's class is over and I'm back home in my chair again, I embrace my tiredness. But just as important, I'm no longer bored. I'm pleased. I triumphed over my body's desire to stay plastered in my chair.

Today I met ten interesting women who are looking for others to go hiking with. I learned some important tips from my classmates that will make me a better hiker. And I'm adding more items to my backpack.

This morning, I faced two non-ideal choices—more of the same setting with guaranteed boredom or pushing against exhaustion and heading to class where I felt I might not be accepted since I wasn't sure that I'd be able to hike.

Instead of what I imagined, I met some great people and was warmly welcomed. One of the leaders told me to come to the first hike which will be a simple out and back three miler on fairly flat terrain. She said if I need to turn around and return, there would be enough leaders for one of them to accompany me back to the trailhead and our parked cars.

Before falling asleep, I smiled and hugged myself. This chemo journey is like hiking through unknown territory. But at least today, out of what I thought were two bad choices, I discovered I chose the best one.

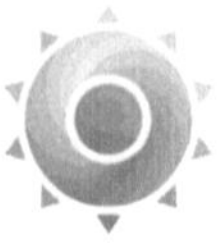

The Side Effects Conundrum

March 25

A MAJOR PART OF CHEMOTHERAPY infusions is managing the body's side effects to each successive treatment. To help tolerate each one I'm instructed to take steroids several days before and after each infusion. My reaction to steroids is high energy, well-being, and insomnia. But to make sure my body doesn't react negatively to each infusion, I also take Benadryl on the day of and several days post each infusion. My side effects from Benadryl are sleepiness, low energy, and exhaustion.

This is where the conundrum begins. I'm taking medicines that cause opposite reactions. For several days I'm both awake and sleepy and simultaneously energetic and depressed. Sigh.

Then my chemo infusions themselves cause their own set of on-going reactions. Following the first infusion session and with each continuing day, my tongue grows more swollen. I've lost taste except for a desire for sweets and salt, have regular headaches that don't go away, and my nose bleeds easily and spontaneously.

The day after each chemo infusion, I receive a shot to increase the production of white blood cells to fortify my compromised immune system so that it can better fight off any future infections. My body's reaction to this shot is similar to getting the flu. It causes me to feel achy and nauseous. I even run a slight fever for a couple of days.

I had been directed by my oncologist to report to her office immediately any new symptoms or side effects from chemo as some reactions can become extremely dangerous. For example, if I ever get a fever over 100, I must immediately go to the emergency room of the nearby hospital.

My lists of new doctors, appointments, tests, and prescriptions grows longer each week as my oncologist's office continues to make referrals to other specialist doctors to try to manage new reactions that surface.

I'm dealing with multiple reactions to each chemo infusion, required medications, follow-up shots. Now I'm adding new side-effect medications for nosebleeds, headache, urinary infections, lost toe nails, and digestion problems.

Some of these extra medications cause diarrhea, others constipation. One even thins my blood which is a risk since I'm already experiencing frequent nosebleeds.

My choice is whether to take each additional medication from specialist doctors to minimize some of these extra side effects of chemo, but then risk dealing with other new side effects created by additional new medication.

Adding more of anything else is like playing Russian Roulette. There is never a medication that doesn't come with new consequences. My one real freedom is saying, *No more! I can live with some discomfort. I don't want more extra doctor visits. No more new medications to merely try to treat another symptom. There is no pain-free life during chemo!*

Acceptance for me brings relief. And simplifying my schedule—with fewer medications to take, fewer additional doctor office visits, and decreased tests—is my new desire for how I want to live now.

I continue each morning marking another big "X" on my hanging wall calendar, which tells me I'm one step closer to the end of chemotherapy.

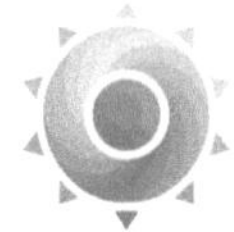

Another Life-Changing Milestone

March 30

THIS MORNING AT 2:30 AM, I received a phone call from my sister Anita. My 100-year-old mother passed quietly in her sleep.

I felt relief that she could leave this world so peacefully. So many aren't given such a gentle exit from this earthly life to whatever comes next.

With father, brother, and now mother gone, her departure makes my two sisters and me the oldest living generation in our family. As one generation passes the torch to the next, I wonder if we've done enough to improve the world and give our children and grandchildren enough support to have good and hopefully better lives.

My older sister by one year, Carol, and her husband, Hugh, were with my mother in Indiana last night while she was falling asleep for the last time. As they gently closed the door to her room, she turned her head in their direction, waved, and sweetly said, "Good-bye."

Most of us wish for the perfect departing scene and phrase. She gifted us with a beautiful one.

The other significance of today? Later this morning is my third chemotherapy infusion. So instead of planning ways to commemorate my mother's life, a different priority requires my attention.

This third one is the first time I'll be going alone without family or friend as my wing person.

Cancer and death are disruptions that refuse to be neatly scheduled for our convenience. Challenges often cling like magnets, stacking one on top of another, indifferent to the weight and eventual overload they cause.

After talking with my sisters immediately after mom's death and reassuring each other that all is well, I knew I needed to fall back asleep and rest my body so that it would be ready for the five-hours of chemicals it would receive later that morning.

I got out of bed, went to the spare bedroom where I picked up and hugged Cinnamon, the big, light-brown teddy bear my mother and family gave me when I turned 40 years old. Then I picked up the family quilt made by my grandmother and headed back to bed.

Surrounded by symbols of love and family, I fell asleep after first sending prayers of love and gratitude to my mother and all departed family who have made sure our lives are filled with support and love.

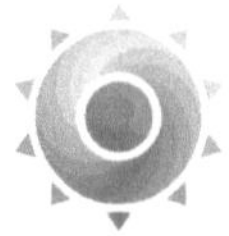

Don't Want to Think of Chemo As Poison But . . .

March 30

ARRIVING AT THE INFUSION CLINIC on my scheduled third chemotherapy date, I'm warmly greeted, ushered to a large lounge chair, and tucked in with warm blankets and multiple pillows.

My nurse and an endless array of other technical and support personnel arrive with friendly smiles, wearing cheerfully themed medical scrubs. They chat with me and check to make sure I have drinks, snacks, and everything I need to be comfortable for the next five hours. I almost feel like I've gone to an expensive spa.

As I'm hooked up to an IV and pumping machine, saline hydration fluids and medicines are started and begin infusing. I lean back in my comfy, overstuffed chair attached to my towering new companion that hums continuously as it works and over the next hours will emit loud alarming beeps whenever it needs attention. Later, when I'll have multiple bags hanging on its hooks and dripping, its alarm can sound loudly every two to five minutes.

In contrast to this initial hour of settling in comfortably, everything changes when it's time for the chemo fluids to flow through the IV port in my arm. My nurse enters wearing an oversized, blue, flowing plastic tent-like coat completely covering her front from her chin to top of her shoes except for where heavy, thick rubber gloves poke through its sleeves. She is accompanied by a second check-nurse standing continuously behind her peering around her shoulder, watching every move to make sure all correct procedures are followed. The cheerful smiles and small talk from earlier are gone. This is serious business.

The first nurse shows the second one each step she's taking. And, the second nurse independently moves in after each action to inspect what's been done by the first. It's clear that what's about to proceed deserves extreme caution and exacting protocol.

I'm shown a six-by-eight-inch plastic bag with lots of black descriptive medical text covering its front. At the top of this bag my nurse points to a long technical name written in large bold letters at the top and asks, "Is this the correct infusion you're supposed to receive?"

I know my oncologist mentioned several weeks ago the medical names of the chemo infusions I would be receiving, but I can only remember them by their short names—

Infusion T and C. On the package she's holding, the easier-to-remember name doesn't appear. Instead, only its formal, long, harder-to-pronounce technical name is present. Since the name on the bag she is holding starts with a T, I nod my head while thinking, *How are patients expected to know?*

Why all these precautions? I wonder. *Why from my previous friendly, chatty, and warm setting is there this sudden shift to an all-serious mode?*

At my last visit before these infusions began, my oncologist explained that even a single drop of chemo infusion liquid on my skin would immediately cause severe burning and damage. *And this is what goes inside me!*

I was instructed after receiving these chemo treatments, to make sure for the next two days to flush the toilet twice after use because I'm discharging toxic chemicals. If I'm urinating toxins, then I quickly surmise that I must be excreting them through saliva and perspiration too—so showering, washing my hair, and changing clothes, bed linens, and towels must be critical as well.

I don't want to think of chemo as poison, but this is a very caustic fluid being fed into my vein that demands serious procedures and precautions.

What's it doing to my body as it flows freely, circulating through my veins, muscles, lungs, and heart? What's happening to my bones, brain, and digestive and nervous systems as it circulates? What kind of extra demand is it placing on my kidneys and liver as they discharge the dying cells and other remnants of the fluids I've received?

The purpose of my chemo infusions is to search out and kill quickly-dividing cells that include any cancerous ones I might still have post-surgery. But sadly, it also kills other rapidly dividing healthy cells, especially those present in my hair, skin, digestive system, and bones.

I know my body's reaction to this kind of chemo includes hair loss, diminished taste, infections from a compromised immune system, crushing exhaustion, and lack of libido. Yesterday, I awakened in the middle of the night with another spontaneous, heavy nosebleed flowing over my face and pillow.

If I stop now and don't continue through to the last scheduled chemo treatment, I'll decrease the benefits of the prescribed program, and that means what I've endured thus far is diminished.

Reluctantly, I proceed saying yes to all four chemo treatments scheduled three weeks apart, spread out over 12 weeks while trying hard not to think that I'm poisoning my body. No mentally healthy person wants to perpetrate such thoughts. And because I know how my mental beliefs affect my body, I try to avoid thinking that way, too.

Daily, I continue to suppress the image of precautions around how caustic my infusion is. Instead, I continue to praise my physical self for being strong like it's always been and say: *You're stronger than any temporary fluid. You know how to survive.*

I welcome the healing vibrations of my home. I walk in nature releasing energy that's not serving me well. I meditate and pray for my body to be strong and welcome offers of similar prayers and healing support from family and friends.

This chemo process is counter intuitive to how I was raised to only eat, drink, and do things that build up my physical body. Destroying healthy cells in the process of eliminating possible cancer-causing ones isn't normal.

I bless the wisdom of my body to endure these 84 days of chemotherapy treatments. When I'm finished, I know my body will build back even stronger again without any subconscious middle-of-the-night fears appearing in dreams or suddenly awakening to threaten me that I still have cancer.

This therapy is to silence and disarm the negative voices and thoughts carried by every cancer survivor. None of us will ever receive an all-clear from medical professionals. When we've finished treatments, we only have the words that we've done all we can to eradicate it, or in some cases merely diminish its presence.

And we are the fortunate ones who, at least, are offered this treatment. Many never get this opportunity.

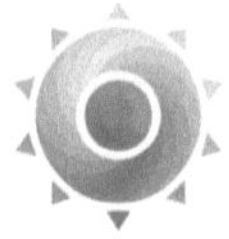

Forest Therapy

March 31

CANCER IS SUCH A WIDESPREAD diagnosis, and locally there are a variety of support groups and activities I can join. At my cancer center last week, I picked up a variety of flyers of activities for people with cancer including Basic Movement Therapy, Art Therapy, Chair Yoga, and Shifting My Perceptions Support Group—just to name several.

The newest flyer titled "Forest Therapy" caught my attention and sent me straight to my browser to learn more. Forest Therapy, also known as forest bathing, originated in Japan, where it's called Shinrin-yoku. In 1982, the Japanese government launched field experiments in 24 forests across the country, comparing participants in urban environments to those in wilderness settings. The results were striking: those in the forest showed lower blood pressure, reduced cortisol levels, slower pulse rates, and more balanced nervous system activity.

That brief bit of research was enough to make me want to attend the upcoming session on the following Thursday at our local park. But when I went to put it on my calendar, I sadly noted that it was on the same day as my third chemotherapy session scheduled earlier in the day. Still, I added it anyway, thinking that it's not the chemo day itself that's the real hurdle, but rather the three to five days that follow it.

Yesterday after chemo infusion number three, I had just enough time in the afternoon to drive to the Forest Therapy session. Arriving at the designated parking lot at Bidwell Park, I opened my car trunk and unpacked my portable folding chair, water bottle, sunhat, and walking shoes. After I joined the gathering of about ten others, the leader guided us away from the normal walking paths into a semi-shaded, tree-free, grassy area. We arranged our chairs in a lopsided circle.

I was relieved that we had only walked a couple hundred yards into the forest. As I carefully unfolded my chair and lowered my body onto its unstable, close-to-the-ground seat, I wondered if this was a good idea, especially with all the new drugs running through my body. But the alternative of going home, sitting in my leather chair all alone, and facing boredom from not having enough energy to do much was less inviting. I stayed.

I was curious about how the leader was going to facilitate this session. We began by introducing ourselves. People gave a wide variety of reasons for coming to the session. Most faced some kind of health challenge or were caseworkers working with people with physical limitations. I mentioned that I was going to spend a lot of time in my chair because I had just had two chemo infusions earlier that day. It was so hot that I had deliberately not worn my wig. Instead, my sunhat clearly signaled that it was covering a bald head.

Our brief introduction to Forest Bathing revealed that it's not just about spending time in the woods. The experience allows us to be immersed in the sights, sounds and smells of the forest. Just as yoga slows down normal movement, Forest Therapy slows down the participant's actions to engage their senses in observing the very subtle being of the forest.

We were instructed to leave our chairs and slowly move outward from our circle into the immediate surrounding areas and notice the forest's movements and sounds.

In my daily solo hikes, I always discovered new things and friendly people. I thought I was learning to know this park well. But I had learned it at a walking pace with a brain busily processing thoughts.

Now I quietly slowed myself to focus on the immediate moment. I led with my eyes, my ears, my nose. It's funny that in this silence I was becoming aware of sounds I didn't normally hear. The humming of flying insects, the fluttering of leaves on the trees around me, the hopping of a bird in the grass nearby. I breathed in the smells of rotting bark and decaying leaves. I watched several small white butterflies or were they moths? Names didn't matter in this sensory focused environment. I observed how they kept within a foot or two of the same area as they flitted from one tall, waving-in-the-wind flower to the next.

As I gently took one step to my left to get out of the direct sun shining in my eyes, I heard a loud crunching sound under my feet. It was simply my shoes breaking some very small sticks and swishing through dried leaves. Life had a different pace. Everything fell into slow motion, punctuated with sounds, then stillness. As soon as I'd zoom in on a small scene and watch it intensely, it would explode with a circus of miniature activities. Actions I'd never noticed before when covering two to five miles on the park's paths. Then distance and what was around the next bend was important. Here, what was within my narrow five foot or less perimeter view was my porthole to experiencing intense activity.

After 15 minutes we were called back to our chairs. I sank into mine, exhausted, and happy to have my body supported again. But as people around the circle shared their experiences, I was lost in my own private world.

It's amazing how an illness can make a person be self-absorbed and isolated from others, even in a group setting. These days that's often how much energy I have. Enough to be with myself. Alone in my own world even when I was in a crowd.

As we folded our chairs, chatted politely with one another, and walked back to our cars, I was more than ready to lie down. But inwardly I was smiling. I'm a tree hugger, a hiker, a lover of nature, and today I discovered a miniature new world I had been missing on my hikes. It reminded me of the first time I went scuba diving and was amazed by the dynamic world found under the surface of oceans and lakes that I had formerly only enjoyed from on top of the water.

At home I tucked myself into my leather chair, covering myself with my favorite multicolored blanket, and fell into a peaceful short sleep.

This is the perfect way to spend the end of a chemotherapy day. I silently sent thanks for the experience that made me appreciate with my eyes, nose, and ears, the fascinating world of woodlands when experienced slowly and patiently.

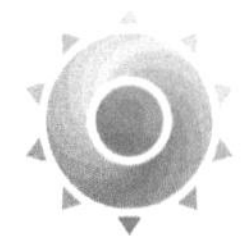

Waves of the Ocean

April 1

Powerful waves surface out of nowhere
without warning.

It's like lying on top a boogie board
floating idly on the ocean's billowing surface.

In the sea around me
waves quietly form and build.
A huge cresting surge grabs my board and accelerates
as it hurtles us both towards shore.

It's useless to turn and fight its momentum.
It's too powerful
All consuming.

Dumped on the beach
Its run spent
Most of the water sucked back.
I wonder at its sparse remnants
lapping gently against my exhausted body
splattered with gritty sand.

After three days of intense steroids
that propelled me upward with energy unleashed,

I face the price of its false highs
with crashing retreat.

Now the Benadryl
that I swallow three days post chemo is in charge.
Overwhelming feelings of listlessness,
sadness, and tears stream silently down my face.
All these as fake as the previous ones of positivity.

Each chemotherapy infusion—
a rollercoaster of accelerating highs
followed by overwhelming lows.
Both surging energy crescendo
and crashing diminuendo
chemically induced.

It's hard when caught up and carried
by these powerful side effects
to know who I truly am.

It's important for me to remember
they're merely coverings
like clothes I wear daily.
Another outer layer to shed, clean, or discard.

Buried deeper inside is my true self,
patiently waiting for recognition that I'm still here.
Ready to be tapped as an endless source of real power
and my own beingness.

Here,
in this center,
I exhale
reconnect
and breathe in the only real
I am.

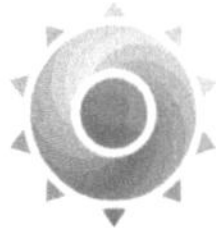

So This is What It's Like to Feel Old

April 2

I AWAKEN FROM SLEEP trying to remember: *Who am I? Where am I?* Mechanically I begin to bend forward as I grasp behind me for my bed's headboard to push my body away from it. Finally sitting upright, I scoot forward several times inching my hips each time closer to the edge of my mattress.

Once there I pause with legs dangling over the side and toes barely touching the floor, while I try to reestablish my bearings and catch my breath.

Unconsciously I begin swinging my upper body back and forth repetitively until I create enough momentum to begin to stand. Almost upright, I exhale hard and reach for my side table for extra support before straining to straighten the rest of the way up.

Again, I search for enough balance to quiet my swaying body and dizzy head.

Taking my first uncertain steps, I hobble as my ankles and feet need time to lubricate and loosen up.

In the bathroom, I hold onto the sink's edge, look in the mirror, and blink several times trying to recognize its reflected image. I'm shocked by the missing long hair replaced by short, sparse, remaining strands. I look like my grandmother when she was 90 years old. I shake my head in disbelief and turn, not wanting more.

As I shuffle off to the kitchen for much needed coffee and breakfast, I feel a heaviness in the back of my throat. Trying to clear it, I utter several loud guttural grunts like those of a barking seal. *This sounds familiar,* I say to myself and search for why.

The memory of my father making similar morning throat-clearing attempts when I was a child of five floats back into my consciousness. Back then I had shuddered, shocked that any human could make such loud, disgusting noises and especially coming from the father I loved so dearly. *Now, these barking sounds belong to me!* I nod and whisper: "Hello, Dad. Now I understand."

This isn't the younger version of myself pre-chemo when I had a swift gait, long-flowing hair, and a loud, clear voice. But this is me now.

On this journey I've learned that how I feel, look, and act can change in an instant. One minute barely existing and the next almost "old-normal."

It's as though I'm in a play and the director keeps throwing me new roles to try out, looking for the one that best suits me at that moment.

So today, old, hobbling, off-balance, throat-clearing Grandma. Tomorrow I'm hoping for rising athlete with terrific balance and overflowing energy as I have a pickleball lesson followed by games with friends.

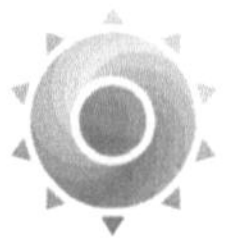

Almost Bald

April 6

NOT ALL KINDS OF CHEMOTHERAPY cause hair loss, but one of the two I'm receiving does.

There are no rules to follow about how to deal with hair loss and approaching baldness from this type of chemo. Some shave their hair off early and even hold parties to celebrate their acceptance and bravery. Others of us hold out until the inevitable finally catches up and leaves us naked without ceremonial shaves.

Even six weeks ago when Joe, my 30-year-old neighbor, found out that I was going through chemo and shaved off his long dreadlocks to support me, I cried tears of gratitude while thanking and hugging him, but kept mine unaltered.

It's funny how I have been shedding hair. First, I lost all my longest hair, then my medium length ones. It makes sense that the longer the hair, the older and more vulnerable it was.

Now my hair is short, and people compliment me on my new haircut. But I haven't cut it. This shorter hair is the younger hair that was hidden amongst all the longer strands. Actually, I like how it looks.

First, I grew it long because of COVID. Then when we were no longer locked down and I could get it styled shorter again, like many others, I thought: *Why bother with the expense? This longer length is easy to maintain.*

Four weeks ago, my sister lovingly offered to shave my head for me before she returned to Southern California. I declined. I wasn't ready. And until about five days ago, I could still be in public without drawing surprised stares from others.

As I undress nightly, I pick numerous blonde hairs off my top, pants, and even socks and throw them in the wastepaper basket by my bed. Daily, I run the vacuum across my floors sucking up the trail I leave everywhere.

Finally, this morning as I looked in the mirror, I clearly saw that my hair no longer looked like it was naturally thin. Now, despite a few scattered, thin, white tufts, it was bare enough to not just shock others, but me as well.

Tonight, when I decided to take an evening walk, I forgot to pull one of my dozens of gifted-from-others caps over my balding head. Outside I recognized an acquaintance walking on the other side of the street. I yelled hello and asked him a question. It was clear by his initial non-response that at first, he didn't recognize me and when he did, he couldn't hide his shock.

I've always wondered what I'd look like as a Buddhist monk. Now, I'm discovering that answer.

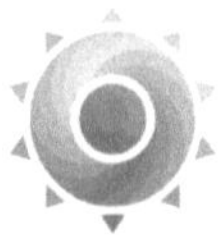

Death Isn't Hidden Anymore

April 7

I REALLY FEEL THE VOLATILITY of life and death as I experience deteriorating changes in my body from chemo. When feeling vibrant and healthy it's easy to ignore the fact that eventually we all die. But when faced with a health crisis like this, it surfaces and confronts me daily.

As I age, I've already noticed gradual declines in my physical and mental abilities. This chemo treatment is showing me how I'll probably be in another 15-20 years.

In the mornings, my movements of getting out of bed and limbering up my stiff body as I move on my way to breakfast mimic almost exactly my mother when she was in her nineties and beyond. When I used to visit her, I needed to remember to slow myself down and allow her extra time to slowly move from one place to another. Now I wish I had been even more patient and unhurried in waiting for her to make her transitions.

It's not just muscles and ligaments that need more time to lubricate and adjust, but also heart to beat more quickly, lungs to send more oxygen to my muscles, and brain to reestablish location and balance.

Although I'm told my health should return after chemo is over—in a year or two from now—there is always the thought in the back of my mind: *What if it doesn't? There's no guarantee it will. I could be like this for the rest of my life.*

But most importantly, with my physical decline, I now imagine I know what it feels like to be 90. And it's not great!

It was a gift watching my mother age. She showed us children, grandchildren, and great grandchildren how to accept declining health with dignity and the ability to adapt and be grateful for what she still had and could do for herself.

As she lost most of her eyesight from macular degeneration, she switched from reading one to two books per week to listening to them on tape. When she finally quit playing organ for group gatherings and services at age 90, she enjoyed not needing to please others with her musical selections and appreciated the extra non-practice time to use for other activities. Five mornings a week she'd do tai chi for 20 minutes moving from standing to sitting exercises as she aged. She relished the weekends when she could skip this self-imposed exercise routine.

I hope her role model is one I can emulate. Now I recognize how brave a person must be to age gracefully and still find ways to appreciate the gift of life.

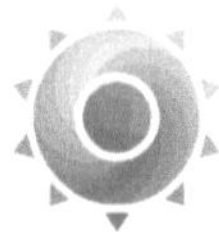

Transition to a Welcome Place

April 8

ANYONE IN PAIN KNOWS the feeling of wanting to escape their body, yet feeling trapped. This morning was one of those times for me. I needed to get out and away—but how to and where to?

When the moment is painful
And my mind's swirling fast,
I stop and remember—
Time to refocus smaller.

I follow my breath
Watching chest rise and fall.

These repetitions
First rough and uncomfortable,
Become slowed and relaxed
as I accept their own rhythm.

Mind softens,
feeling deeper into my center
Here's where peace resides

One single breath at a time,
with no hurry to the next.

Eyes fall shut,
lift upwards in darkness
In this blank setting my brain rests.

What comes next?
Peace?
Sleep?
It does not matter.

I've been transported
to a more welcome place.

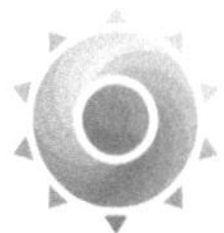

Brain Fog—My New Excuse

April 9

WHAT'S HAPPENING TO MY short-term memory? I always wondered if I would get chemo brain. *But do I have it now?*

My morning breakfast is simple. It's just coffee with cream and two soft scrambled eggs. I don't prepare them in a specific order. I just start somewhere and continue until I'm ready to carry my plate of cooked eggs and full cup of coffee into the front room where I eat in my chair and catch up on the daily news.

This morning after making my eggs I thought I had forgotten to make my coffee. I reached up into the cupboard, pulled down the coffee canister, and took out the measuring cup to get filtered water from the refrigerator. But when I opened the top of the coffee maker to fill its strainer with ground coffee beans, there were wet, hot grounds already there. Confused, I looked around the kitchen. On the counter by the door to the front room sat a steaming cup of coffee. I hadn't forgotten to make it, merely that I had.

I shook my head. I had zero recall of preparing it. *How could I forget something so recent, so routine?*

Lately, while playing pickleball, when a foul is made, I often can't remember who was serving or what's the score. So, I helplessly pick up the ball after the rally is over and don't know who to throw it to. Similarly, when I serve and need to call out the score, I can't remember what it is and ask my partner for help.

Thankfully, on my good days, I can still play almost as well as I could pre-chemo. Yes, I tire more easily and need to sit out games more often after completing several. But serving the ball and returning it, I'm still fine since these actions take place in the present and don't require recall of what happened moments earlier.

Everyone—especially those my age—complains about short-term memory forgetfulness. But now I have a new excuse other than age. I simply blame these memory glitches on chemo brain.

It's nice to have a non-age-related excuse. I wonder, *How long I can continue to use it after chemo is over?*

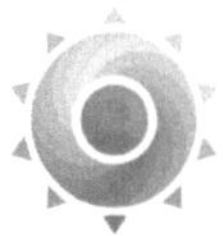

Where Does My Face Stop?

April 10

LAST NIGHT ON DAY 54 of chemo, I finally shaved my head. It was time to enter this next hairless stage with dignity. I had seen enough men wearing ridiculous comb overs to not try any longer to pretend that my almost hairless head wasn't a bigger eye catcher than just being cleanly shaven and bald.

This morning, I had a social meeting and wanted to get ready for it.

After putting on my hearing aids, I realized that they are no longer cleverly disguised, nestled under my hair, and out of sight. Now they rest on top of each ear clearly exposed. And without hair around them, they sit more vulnerable, easier to bump off. *I'll have to be more careful.*

Starting with facial cream, I wonder: *Where does the face end?* I hesitate and then put it all over my face and bare head, too. *Why not? These cells need moisturizer and nutrients too.*

Applying make-up, I feel as though every layer is exposed. I was taught when putting on blush to brush it across my cheek bones back to my hairline. *But there is no hairline, so where do I stop my brush stroke? Do I just continue the whole way around my head?*

And what about the darker blush I always brush on my upper forehead to recede its length into the background a bit? *Where does the forehead stop?*

My lipstick is now much too bright as suddenly it is front and center without hair on the sides of my face to balance its color. The same is true for eyeliner on eyes that have no eyelashes or eyebrows. I look like the five-year-old who is playing with her mother's makeup, and it's too much color on her young, innocent face.

With such fair skin my never-been-tanned, shockingly light-colored head is bright white. I feel like the top end of a Q-tip. As I try on hats and earrings, I think: *Here is where I can add some color.* With a hat and large dangling earrings, I add distracting drama to draw attention away from my face.

I decide that I'll wear the head coverings when I'm outside. But most of the time at home, I'm going to go bare headed. I've always hated hats or wearing anything on my head. Even when I lived back East in snowy, cold weather, I'd only wear earmuffs and never a hat.

As I sit in my chair and begin rubbing my hands freely over my formerly shedding head, it's scratchy from shaving. But as I do this, I realize a new freedom of willfully touching my scalp again. I couldn't do this for the past seven weeks because any touch or rubbing increased hair fall out.

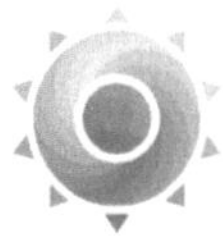

Rodrigo and Cancer

April 11

TODAY MY GODSON, who is as close to me as a grandson, called me. I was delighted when I picked up my ringing phone to see that it was Rodrigo calling. Immediately I swiped the FaceTime answer bar on my phone and clicked on the video view, excited about getting to see and spend time with him.

Rodrigo's young seven-year-old face lit up my screen. His immediate reaction was a loud gasp and a look of utter surprise as he raised his phone-free hand to cover his open mouth. Wide-eyed and deeply concerned, he quickly added, "But Goma, you…you look beautiful!"

I knew he was embarrassed by his initial reaction to my completely bald head and tired, drawn face. I laughed and responded, "Don't be embarrassed by your surprised reaction. Guess what I think every time I look in a mirror?

Who is that strange looking woman? It can't be me. And I know that I don't look like the Goma you expected, do I?"

After talking a little bit longer about how different I look and how, one day at a time, I'm making it through these chemo treatments, my iPhone screen began filling up with funny characters popping up over his image, as his face turned into a blue talking monkey, then a pink pig followed by a dinosaur. I join in the fun, threatening to hang up on him if he didn't return to the good-looking godson I love. With this teasing we were back to our normal interactions, laughing and playing with our phones as we talked.

During this call and our previous ones, I hope my godson learns that even though a person can look different when they're facing a difficult health challenge, they still are the person he knows and loves.

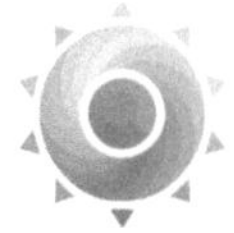

Support Group & New Cancer Perspective

April 12

DURING MY PREVIOUS two breast cancer episodes, it was easy for me to say, *I don't need to join support groups.* These previous cancers, when diagnosed, were still in an early Stage 1, and all of the cancer was easily removed by simple lumpectomy surgeries.

But now, I'm in a new city and don't have local family or deep friendships for support. My cancer medical center offers a variety of activities. I decide to join their monthly in-person support group and a second online one.

This time, I've decided to make my journey a time of healing and personal growth. I've already resolved to quit trying to be a superwoman, admit my vulnerability, and take advantage of the chance to speak with others facing cancer in a therapeutic setting.

It's nice to finally be able to talk with people who understand about exhaustion, fear, loneliness, medication side effects, pain, and the list goes on. Here is a place where few or many words can be spoken, immediately grasped, and always accepted.

How many different words are there for compassion, admiration, and awe? I need them all to describe the people I meet in these groups. They include some of the bravest people I've ever encountered.

Although my current cancer and chemotherapy are major disrupting events in my life and health, what I'm facing is so much less than the experiences some in these groups face. I hear and see how hard cancer and its treatments are for many.

My four chemo infusions are extended over in 15 weeks. Although they're dramatic to me, mine are a mere blip on the radar screen compared to those with more serious stages and forms of cancer. One has been receiving chemo off and on, for over eight years. Another gets treatments weekly all year long.

A few have maxed out and chemo is either no longer an option or on their own they have said, "No more."

I've been self-absorbed in my cancer journey. It's life changing and dramatic for me. But I can only imagine the extra burdens others face with cancers much different and more advanced than my own. With my infusions, I'm only hoping to destroy any remaining cancer cells not removed during surgery. My cancer was localized in three small lumps that were easily extracted. But others face infusions hoping to merely slow cancer's rapid spread or have a better quality of life, for just a bit longer.

I'm amazed by the collective intelligence that many in my support groups have gained. They realize that cancer isn't all of who they are. A few even say simply that if they must face an end to life, they are ready for what's next.

My medical bills are mostly covered by Medicare and medical supplemental insurance pays the rest. I am retired and no longer need to work. My retirement pays my other necessary bills. But many others in these groups need to keep working through their illness. They have children to raise or are caregivers to parents that count on their incomes. Mounting financial burdens often drive their decisions about treatments or continuing to go to work. The mounting additional burdens they face, beyond cancer and treatments, make my life sound like a vacation at a resort.

During these sessions, we share an hour to just be ourselves and enjoy the comfort of being with others who understand.

Our facilitator chooses different topics for each week. This week we discussed how to live with pain. The insights and personal experiences about how to cope with pain and continue to live life are remarkable.

This support group reminds me that I belong to a community much larger than myself. During our sessions, I feel a tremendous flow of love and support, finding comfort among others on this same journey. It is often easier to learn from those living with cancer than from experts who only cite statistics and studies. Collectively, regardless of our diagnosis, we are bright, beautiful people.

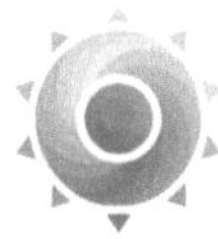

No Longer Invisible

April 15

HAVING LIVED IN BIG CITIES including New York, Philadelphia, Washington, D.C., and San Diego, I am used to not thinking about how I look when I run to the store or walk aimlessly through neighborhood streets. After all, in large metropolitan areas there are so many people that you can spend a whole day and not recognize anyone. It is easy to fade into the background and be invisible, because other truly unusual, interesting-looking people are everywhere.

I remember one Halloween years ago walking down my neighborhood street several blocks off Time Square in New York City. I passed two people obviously headed to a Halloween party dressed up to look like frightening monsters. After they passed me, I laughed thinking to myself: *If you think you're scary, you should have seen the man I passed a couple of blocks back who wasn't headed to any party.*

Now I live in a middle-sized town of around 105,000 residents. Here most people look similar to one another. It's not uncommon for us to wave at someone thinking we know them and then as we get closer realize they're not who we thought they were. When we make such a mistake, we laugh and end up talking with each other anyway, saying we're sure we'd become friends if we only took the time to learn more about each other.

As I began to lose my hair one of my daughters immediately had fun buying and sending me hats. Local friends also gifted me others. The cancer center director, where I go for treatments, hauled out a box and said, "Choose one."

When I still had some hair peeping out in the front and under the sides of my hats, I didn't look unusual. But as I became completely bald, the hats no longer looked normal. Cancer caps are meant to cover the whole head and not just sit on top with hair flowing somewhere below. There are even styles called "cancer hats."

Now, when I wear my hats on my bare head in public, it's more obvious to others that I don't have hair.

It's become common for strangers to come up to me and offer comments about my cancer without even asking if I have it. My appearance says it all. One person reassured me that there was life after chemo. Another said she had walked in my shoes and knew what I was facing. Other people merely stare too hard and long or ask about how I am feeling.

I know these people mean well when they approach me in public. My problem is that *I'm more than cancer*. When

I finally have enough energy to go out in public to shop or run errands, I'm not thinking about having cancer. I'm just Linda doing her daily chores. It's a necessary relief to forget and have a break from the cancer parts of my life.

So, when people look at me funny or want to talk to me about what I'm going through, I'm once again pulled back into a cancer world.

I love how warm and friendly most people are. But if you see a person going through a health challenge, remember they are more than their body. Greet them and talk about anything other than health. And even if you think you've navigated their situation, remember that's your history and not theirs.

The last thing we need to hear about is someone else's cancer story. We're already overflowing with our own experiences. And we're overloaded with advice and treatments from our many doctors and specialists.

Wait and see if we bring it up or if we ask for advice about your experience. Sometimes we may be ready for such conversations. Otherwise, allow us the freedom from the one aspect of our lives that we can't hide and is not open for public discussion.

I feel a bit like the very pregnant woman who strangers want to pat her stomach or ask when she's due. Or the person with the black eye or walking on crutches with a cast on their foot. How many times must they explain themselves to others and especially to people they don't even know.

We all need to be more than just our bodies. And many times, we crave the privilege of being hidden in a crowd.

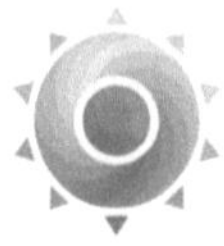

Freedoms of No Hair

April 18

AS I ADJUST TO THE HUGE changes that come with having no hair left on my body anywhere, I laugh as I notice many new advantages of being totally hairless. Today I decided to focus not on what I've lost, but on what I've gained. Here are some of the benefits I came up with.

- **Mornings, getting dressed is faster** as there is no hair to brush and style. It's nice having this extra time to enjoy my breakfast at a more leisurely pace.
- **My bathroom shower feels spacious** as I no longer have shampoos, hair conditioners, razer, and shaving cream cluttering shelves. Similarly, my bathroom vanity and drawers have more room, as I've packed away all hair-related paraphernalia.

- **Only one towel** is needed when I bathe or shower as a second one isn't needed to wrap my dripping hair up into it while I dry off my body with the second one.
- **Restaurant outdoor misters don't ruin my hair.** Sitting with friends outside during happy hour in the heat of summer, misters above often begin spraying to cool us off. My first reaction is: *Oh no, my hair will go straight!* But there's no hair to lose its curl. Now I just enjoy the cooling droplets and smile.
- **My hair doesn't slap my face and hurt** when I roll my windows down in my moving car. Instead, I enjoy the wind's full force for the first time without covering my hair in a scarf or tying it back from my face. It's that same type of freedom we used to enjoy on bicycles before helmet rules became mandated.
- **My purse is a bit lighter and roomier** without a hairbrush, clips, and supplies. It's also easier to find what I'm looking for in its more spacious interior.
- **I take extra showers any time I want** without worrying that the steam will ruin my hair style. Also, showering time is lessened without hair to wash, conditioners to apply to untangle my hair, and legs to shave.
- **Walking bareheaded in the rain without an umbrella or rain hat**, I join many other hairless souls on the streets without worries about our hair getting drenched.
- **No need to brush hair off clothes**. I'm so used to picking long hairs off my clothes. **Now I can even wear black tops** and not worry about long blonde strands decorating their surface.

- **My house stays cleaner** now that there is no hair to vacuum up from floors or collect off of furniture.
- **I can use a smaller suitcase when I travel**, now that there's no need for a hair dryer, brushes, shampoos, conditioners, gels, shower cap, and accompanying styling paraphernalia.
- **I no longer need to shave my legs**, and they are always smoother than ever. The same could be said about my eyebrows that no longer need plucking or trimming as they are completely gone, too. Being hairless everywhere has its advantages.

There are advantages to this new chapter of my life. And it's not all bad!

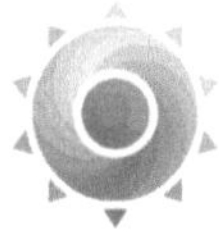

Last Chemo—But Not Celebrating Yet

April 19

I REMEMBER THE FIRST TIME I bicycled a century (100-mile distance) along with hundreds of others on the Eastern Shore of Maryland. As I crossed the finish line, I was greeted by my cheering husband and daughter waving their arms wildly in the air. I wasn't calling out to them and celebrating as I rode up beside them. I burst into tears. My waiting family was confused. This was not the finish they had imagined sharing with me.

Inside myself I was relieved and happy, but there were so many pent-up emotions I hadn't expressed. Feelings I'd been holding back for too many miles while I wondered if I could complete even the next mile let alone this whole difficult century. Before that ride, my longest bicycling distance was only 50 miles. So, doubling it was a huge accomplishment for me. I was bursting with pride about what I had accomplished but first tears of relief and then cheers of celebration.

Today was my fourth and last infusion. This morning, I crossed off day 84 on the calendar hanging on my bathroom wall knowing that this was the last chemo treatment I'd be receiving.

I went to this infusion session alone since it was only a mile away and on the treatment days, I always felt strong enough to drive myself there.

To everyone's surprise inside the medical center, I wasn't ready to celebrate this final milestone. I knew too well that this last infusion wasn't the real end.

After this treatment I hadn't planned a party with friends at the infusion center where it's customary for the person completing their infusion therapy to walk out into the serenity garden and hit the tall Japanese two-foot long rectangular bell. Most people invite friends and family to join them in this garden bell-ringing celebration. I not only didn't invite anyone. My few new local friends didn't even know the date of this last infusion.

Today after new chemicals dripped into my body for five hours, I knew the hell I'd be facing in the following four days. And it would be weeks and months after that before my body could slowly start the long trudge up the steep mountain of rebuilding health.

Infusion days themselves had been non-eventful as I was still on steroids that created lots of energy. I never really felt the downsides until two days after each treatment. I dreaded those days. I was so done with the escalating and more difficult symptoms of each successive infusion, that I seriously think if my oncologist had prescribed a fifth one, I might have said, *No more!*

Medical professionals don't tell new patients beginning chemo that it's not uncommon for people to max out part way through and just quit. For some types of cancer, I've heard that the quit rate can be higher than 25%.

In my cancer support groups there were several who hit this point and said, "I'm going to heal another way." Or, "I was only doing this for my children, not myself. I can't continue to please them. I can't do it any longer."

These past three weeks following the third infusion, my body has been less able and willing to hike and play pickleball. I still try to do some daily physical activities since research shows that exercise helps diminish the side effects of chemo. But my will power isn't as strong as it once was.

There is nothing new or exciting to discover about this journey. My body has continued its decline, dragging my emotions and spirit with it. I have weeks ahead where this fourth dose will run through my body destroying more healthy cells and hopefully any final remaining cancerous ones still around.

My celebration is only that this is the last chemo infusion. I'll have completed all that were prescribed for my tumor type and stage of cancer.

As my chemo session ends and I am ready to leave the clinic, I am surprised by an announcement that all medical staff not doing critical work with patients, are being called away from their posts. Twelve of us walk out into the garden. I am handed a gong hammer and realize I have need to do something.

I smile and thank everyone for being so supportive of me and others receiving treatments under their care. I acknowledge the privilege of striking this bell with my mallet. I turn, hit it, they clap and cheer. A few photos are taken with my phone, and we walk back inside so I can be discharged.

I'll text the photos to family and friends who have been supporting me long distance from across the USA and Canada. I always choose ones of me smiling and looking happy, so they won't worry.

Now off to do errands like getting food and supplies for the days and weeks ahead when I won't have the energy or feel as strong.

It's good to have finished this part of the chemo race.

A few tears flow down my face once I'm finally alone in my car. But this century marathon still has more miles before it's completed.

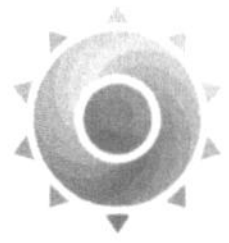

Mindful of Small Moments

April 21

SITTING AGAIN THIS MORNING in my well-seasoned chair, I'm tired of the all–too–familiar post infusion let down.

This repetitious routine of feeling tired, achy, disoriented, and bored has become well known and unwelcome.

For the past 20 years, I've been studying and practicing mindfulness meditation. I've learned that when we think about the past, we can easily experience regrets. And when we go to the future, we can be filled with fears triggered by the "what ifs?" The only safe place is found in the immediate present now.

After the death of my husband, one way I got through the early difficult days as a widow was by asking myself, *"Am I okay right now? Right now, as in this very narrow second of time?"* I'd continue this inner dialogue by reminding myself that Bill and I never spent every moment of each day together. We both led active lives. I traveled with my work and was sometimes gone for a week at a time. We'd missed each other when separated, but we'd function well and weren't miserable.

Crying when I missed him after his death, I discovered that the tears were propelled by my inner dialog about events in the past that I should have appreciated more or in the future about things he'd miss. But when I used my mindfulness training and redirected my mind to come to the present moment and my inner dialogue focused only on the now moment, my tears would stop abruptly without the necessary fuel about the past or future to keep them going.

Sometimes the present moment must get very short. By that I mean not thinking about the whole breath as I breathed in or out. Only feeling and experiencing the small fragment in a single breath.

Discontent with the despair my chemo-infused body kept producing, I knew something had to change. But I couldn't escape my unhappy body. Again, I wished I could but didn't know how.

Instead, I focused on slicing this present moment as thinly as I could.

As my mind became quiet and I observed small bits of this "now" moment, I recognized different and new sensations that were also present. My front door was open. As I sat focused on the present, I felt the most beautiful wisp of spring breeze caressing my cheek. My line of sight as my head tilted upwards included the gently swaying branches of the old walnut tree outside my window. I laughed as I noticed two squirrels chasing each other, leaping from limb to limb in their simple, endless game of tag.

The softness of the leather cushioned my hands resting on the arms of my chair.

I shut my eyes as my brain slowed down like a swing that's no longer pushed and then rests still in silent darkness that is so familiar.

This gift of peace is one I had lost as I became consumed by my treatments and responses to chemo. This present space was greater than any smaller parts of me.

I had forgotten this place of respite.

I relaxed and felt truly at home.

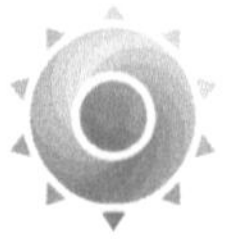

My Energy Bank

May 15

NOW THREE WEEKS AFTER my last chemo, my body is officially finished with infusion treatments. My oncologist says my energy should substantially return in another month or so. I hope she's right because the fourth and last treatment made it considerably more difficult to maintain doing more than the absolute minimum each day. I'm embarrassed to say that the TV is my constant entertainment most of the day, and I don't care about the quality of its programs because I doze off continuously.

For so many years in the business world, we thought that time management was a critical skill to teach people. But time is what I have too much of now. Post-chemo (it's fun to finally say those words) what I'm finding is the need to manage my energy. Wanting to build my body up again, I've signed up to take several 3–5-mile hikes and joined a new pickleball league. These commitments force me out of the house and to become physically active again.

I'm finding that I can do these types of activities again, but after each, I'm back in my chair resting, sleeping, and recuperating.

Two weeks ago, my average recovery time after a three-hour activity was 24 hours. Now it's closer to 12 hours unless I've added too many extra small errands afterwards.

On my phone calendar, when I schedule anything, I immediately block out necessary recovery time. Exercise, for example, takes more recuperation time than lunch with friends. But after all activities, I'm back resting in my chair.

When I ignore or forget this scheduling trick, my body lets me know I've gone too far. Wherever I am, it's as though a gray curtain descends over my face, and I'm ready to sleep wherever I am. Even the unswept, concrete sidewalk downtown this morning looked comfortable. My friends when they see this change suddenly grow concerned.

As much as I want to return to a normal life, treating my energy as a treasured commodity is part of that process.

I guess learning to become patient with my body's return to health is another skill I'm being forced to develop. The consequences of not pacing myself are too expensive.

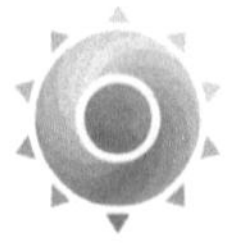

What Now?

June 1

FOR THE PAST YEAR the top priority in my life has been cancer and its endless activities.

Now, after this last chemo infusion, I am suddenly left with a single activity—an every-eight-weeks oncology checkup appointment. I'm finally through with placing cancer first and solely in my life. My schedule now that chemotherapy is over is empty, wide open, filled with nothing. I stare at my blank calendar for this month and then look at the following months. There is only one medical appointment. *What now?*

I'm left with empty spaces to fill in my life. I'm now facing the post-cancer treatment life that every person who has ever had cancer dreams about. Except for a once-a-day pill, which keeps my body from producing the hormones my cancer needs to exist, and regular oncologist appointments to monitor the drug side effects and my overall health, I'm done with medical routines.

It's so sudden. Unfamiliar. A transition to be sure. *But to what next?*

I should be celebrating. I should be happy. I should be quickly filling my calendar with all sorts of fun things. Instead, this morning I sit here stumped— trying to remember how I used to live and wondering if that's even what I want again.

I've changed. This Linda is different from the Linda of a year ago.

I'm no longer as unconscious about the fact that life on this earthly plane doesn't go on forever. I've opened my heart towards the suffering of myself and others. I've found soothing healing in simple things, like watching squirrels out my window, rejoicing as my taste slowly returns making food more exciting, and feeling gentle morning breezes.

People think that I've finally returned to my former life. But what they are expecting is the old pre-cancer Linda. *But am I her?* I find myself in confusion asking, *Who is this new post-cancer person?*

It's like taking all your furniture out of a room so you can renovate it. Now that it's repainted, with different flooring and curtains, you ask, "How much of my old stuff belongs in this new room?" Some of the old needs to be tossed. Other pieces cleaned and refurbished. And with this new arrangement what needs to be added?

When I ask, *What now?* the answers aren't obvious. I need time to get to know this new person. Time without non-essential obligations.

As I begin to appear at previous activities and groups, people are excited by my return. I enjoy seeing familiar faces I've not seen for a while. I've been asked to consider being on a board of directors position for a local non-profit organization and asked to consider being president of a local social organization.

I know enough about myself that these positions would consume me. I politely reply to each offer, "I'm taking a year off from new obligations. I need time for myself."

To be honest, the treatments may be over, but my energy isn't back to normal. I'm still healing on the inside even though I look normal on the outside.

This is truly a time of self-reinvention, self-redefinition, and self-nurturing that can't be rushed. I need time to let this slowly evolve.

Before me are so many possibilities. But running quickly after the first few doesn't feel right. What I'm enjoying most is sitting, thinking, and writing about whatever comes up in the moment.

I also enjoy the simple rhythm of the garden. I'll stroll outside to dig, first crouching low to see more clearly, then sinking down until my knees are planted in the earth. There is a quiet satisfaction in getting my fingernails dirty as I uncover and nurture each plant. This allows me time to be still and see what arises in the moment, breathing in the scent of blossoms, damp soil, and decaying leaves.

Slowly I explore beginning thoughts about my question *What Now?* I know if I don't immediately engage with the first thoughts, other more developed ones will come if I wait patiently and enjoy exploring my new life.

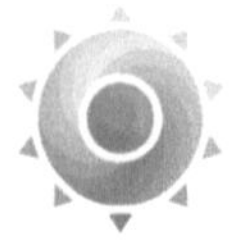

Futility of Predictions

June 20

WE ALL HEAR STORIES about people who go through chemotherapy infusions for cancer and are still able to work full time while receiving treatments. Doctors and the medical community often share these examples when we ask what it will be like once our treatments start.

The problem with these positive examples is, as both doctors and cancer patients know well, everyone is a study of one. Just because some experience particular effects doesn't mean we all will. Also, there are many types of chemotherapy, making it impossible to predict what any specific experience will be like.

The stories about others working full time made me feel like I was a wimp on the five days surrounding each infusion. On those days I wouldn't have been well enough to go to my job if I were still employed.

And friends, people who hiked and played pickleball with me, and neighbors who saw me mowing my lawn all thought I was doing spectacularly. What they didn't see was the Linda post-exercise, crashed on the couch—exhausted without energy to cook even a simple meal. Following all strenuous activities (and the word "strenuous" got redefined downward after each successive treatment), I crashed and slept. During these recovery times no one saw me. So, it wasn't a part of the picture people held and told others about when relating how I was doing.

After my first breast cancer in 2011 and the publication of my first book, *Blind Curves: One Woman's Unusual Journey to Answer What Now?,* in 2013, I was invited to be the keynote speaker on a breast cancer survivors' cruise sponsored by *Breast Cancer Wellness* magazine. On this cruise, I met hundreds of other breast cancer survivors and had time during the six-day cruise to hear many first-hand conversations about their journeys through radiation and chemotherapy. Many of these women had worked during their treatments because they needed the income to support their children, themselves, and even their parents.

But most women who continued working also said that the moment they got home, they headed to their couch or bed to crash. And most maxed out their sick and personal leaves during their worst treatment days and for their plethora of doctor visits and treatment appointments.

Having consulted with large companies most of my career, I've heard heart-felt stories from co-workers of people with cancer about how they've covered in the workplace for their peers going through chemotherapies by doing some of their work and lightening their assignments.

We all truly are stories of one when we go through treatments. What others and even doctors don't see is what we experience when we're out of the public scrutiny and view.

I felt that something was wrong with my self-motivation when I couldn't live up to the references by those medical professionals who claimed that many patients maintain their normal routines during radiation and chemo.

And as much as I criticize doctors and the medical community for their sometimes difficult-to-live-up-to examples, we the patients are the ones who are persistent in our demands for predictions about what we will experience.

I was probably one of the most insistent ones wanting answers because I needed to know them before I said yes to any treatments. Living alone, I wanted to know if I'd be able to take care of myself or would need to hire outside help.

And now, I'm the same person saying that expert opinion is what makes me feel bad when I now fall short of it. I shouldn't both demand predictions and then fault them.

Going through difficult cancer treatments has left me feeling powerless at times. The more I learn about my cancer and the treatments I am receiving, the more in control I feel about a life I've lost the ability to navigate.

We, the people with cancer, often have created false impressions and others believed it and spread incomplete stories about how well we're doing or not doing. Sigh. I'm at fault for both.

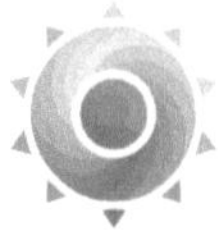

Time to Think & Dig Deeper

July 21

INITIALLY CANCER CAN be an acceptable excuse we give others for stepping back from some of our current and future obligations and activities. But as our treatments progress and our energy decreases, it moves from an excuse to a necessity to eliminate all non-essential endeavors.

Stripped of life's usual distractions—projects, social engagements, obligations to work, family, friends, and community—I found myself alone with time to think. I asked: *Who am I beneath all these activities that usually fill my days? Without them, what's left of me?*

My search for answers isn't unique to me and many others facing cancer. There are many other great life disruptors like failed relationships, loss of people we love, financial setbacks, or other kinds of life crises. Incidences where we're forced to move deeper through our outer layers of distractions and protection. In such times I find I'm living a life that no longer makes sense.

Cancer for me is a time when my memorized answers to life's toughest questions are being rebirthed and retested. I'm forced daily to go deeper into the meanings of who I am when I look at three separate parts of me—my physical body, mind, and emotions.

Although my physical body can be demanding, limit my mobility, and distract me with its distress signals, *it's not who I really am.*

With cancer I've been through three major surgeries. Each time a portion of my body was cut out and the remaining tissues reorganized. And this time chemotherapy's use of infusions to kill off rapidly dividing cells has stressed my body to its limit and produced side effects that are so vocal and debilitating that my physical body often demands my total attention. But I've kept remembering and relearning more deeply my established belief that *I am not my body!*

During this cancer journey, I've relearned, *I'm not my constant running thoughts and mind.* Pain and discomfort cause me to over analyze what's happening and come up with endless dialogues about what to do. Although some of this thinking is productive, much of its endless chatter is useless, repetitive noise. Again, I keep reminding myself, *I am more than my thoughts.* And when I need a break, I relax and quit feeding it with energy, attention, and demands for solutions.

And finally, *I'm more than my emotions,* although to live life fully, it's necessary to feel, process, and express them. But with cancer disrupting much of my life and threatening my physical and mental health, I have to be able to both give my emotions a voice and then turn them off to get a chance to rest, heal, and look for joy found within the limits of my current state.

What I'm relearning at a much deeper level is I am more than my physical body, my thoughts, and my emotions.

I am the deeper soul or spirit that existed before I was born, is with me now, and will continue after my death.

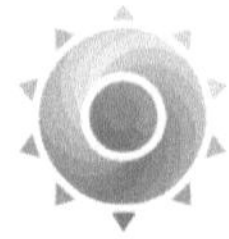

Shocked by Compliments from Strangers

August 15

SHOPPING AT THE LOCAL Safeway last night, I pushed my heavy cart with a front wheel that wouldn't spin correctly toward the self-check-out when a young woman in her early twenties approached me.

"I hope you don't mind my saying this . . . and . . . I don't mean to be intrusive, but you have the most beautifully shaped head."

Then she quickly added, "And I love your shaved haircut."

I'd never dreamed that the shape of my head could be something that others would notice—let alone compliment me about it. Up until four months ago it was hidden under my long, fluffy hair. I know I didn't hide my surprise well as

I raised my eyebrows and pulled my head back slightly. But then I quickly corrected myself.

"What a nice compliment. Thank you."

We smiled at each other and continued to complete our shopping. It's strange, but suddenly I held my head higher off my shoulders, and my cart felt lighter and easier to steer.

This chemo journey has been full of surprises. But this one really caught me off guard. Here, I'm still hoping that I don't draw stares for looking like a cancer patient—especially since I refuse to wear a head covering over my very short hair in public anymore. Instead, tonight I'm gifted with a compliment from a stranger who needed to express her admiration for how I look.

This isn't the only admiring comment I've drawn in recent weeks. Several nights ago, I went to an outdoor concert. As I waited in line to buy a beverage, an attractive young man approached me and asked:

"Did you shave your hair yourself or get a barber to do it for you? You look great!"

OMG is all I could think. Suddenly people think I'm hip and admire an older woman who keeps up with the trends with a shaved head.

I smiled and said:

"Did it myself, and thanks for the compliment."

When I speak to audiences about how people handle change, I explain how we first notice what we're losing before we see what we gain. Well, I've certainly noted the many losses I've experienced through this cancer journey. But I've also seen some positives as I got deeper into the treatment and afterwards in recovery.

Now I'm noticing even more unexpected gifts, and I'm having fun with my weekly changes in appearance as my hair grows a bit longer each month, and my eyelashes and eyebrows are slowly returning.

Friends my age tell me, "Keep this close-shaved look. You've always been a bit edgy, and this style suits you. It makes you look much younger than your age."

Now I have choices about how I want to appear. But I'm going to let my hair continue to grow. I'm curious. *Will it get curly when it's longer like so many post-chemo people experience?*

Once it's shoulder length I can decide if I want to return to this close-shaven look or enjoy my longer hair. It's nice to be in charge and have choices again.

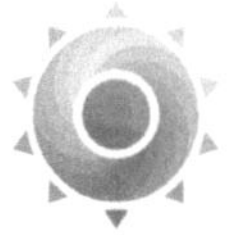

Third Time's Not the Charm

August 31

TODAY IS THE ANNIVERSARY of my appointment a year ago with my breast surgeon when she looked at me sternly, forehead furrowed, and eyebrows raised as she spoke the words neither of us wanted to hear.

"Linda, you have cancer again. And yes, it's early stage, but this time there are three small tumors, and we know this type is aggressive."

This certainly wasn't the birthday present I was hoping for on that day, but cancer ignores birthdates, anniversaries, and holidays.

I wasn't shocked by her words. After all, I'd heard them twice before in my life. Listening to this now familiar news yet a third time, I felt as if its raw edges had been worn down.

"Oh," I simply said, familiar with what I expected the road ahead to look like—needle biopsy, sonogram, MRI, mammography, surgery, healing, and lots more.

I knew two weeks earlier when I found the familiar feeling of a small lump in my right breast, in practically the same location where breast cancer appeared the year before, that there was a strong probability cancer was repeating itself. But there was the hope I was simply feeling scar tissue from last year's surgery, even if this felt more pronounced than it should have been. That's the advantage of doing your own self-exams. I had found my previous two breast cancers through similar monthly checks. When you do it monthly, it's easier to recognize subtle differences.

After hearing her words, they felt so normal that I wanted to lean forward and console my doctor who appeared to be taking this news harder than I was.

"This time," she continued, "we'll need to take more tissue from your right breast and be much more aggressive. You'll be left with half of your breast gone. Your nipple will point sideways rather than forward."

I nodded.

"I give up. Take what you need, and I'll live with an uneven profile. Why should it matter?"

She wanted to talk about the possibilities of inserting an artificial implant. But that would need to be removed and replaced surgically with a replacement in 15-20 years. I didn't want to think about cosmetic surgery in my nineties. I know many people don't live that long, but my mother lived to 100, so I have the genes for longevity.

My breast surgeon didn't want me to live with a deformed body that reminded me daily of another cancer surgery. She told me about another possibility. I was an ideal candidate for transferring belly fat along with an artery and vein to my breast after a mastectomy had been performed. After this surgery I would look normal again except for the new scars.

Now a year later, I look back and realize I had no idea about the difficulties ahead. Sometimes not being able to see the future is a blessing. Because one day at a time I've made it through. It would have been much harder if I had known that I'd have to wait three and a half months to coordinate the dates of the possible hospitals, two surgeons (cancer and plastic), and operating room for the surgery. Even more challenges would come when I had finally recovered eight weeks after the surgery.

In the follow-up post-surgery visit in December, I was told by both surgeons that all three lymph nodes removed during the mastectomy were cancer free. Moving abdominal tissue to my breast and reconnecting a vein and artery with my own transplant had been successful. My plastic surgeon assured me that in a year, the small triangular scar on my right breast would fade and I'd look normal. And most importantly both surgeons guaranteed that they had removed all the cancer in the breast and surrounding areas. So, we all thought I was cancer free.

Finally, I was planning my post-cancer life, filling my calendar with social events, hikes, and ways to meet as many people as I could in my new town. For the first time since August, I no longer had to worry about picking up an infection like COVID, flu, or RSV that would have delayed my surgery.

I had one last post-surgery medical appointment in February to see my oncologist. I assumed I'd get a new prescription for hormone suppression medicine to take for the next five years. Entering her office, I was looking forward to having this third cancer event behind me.

Instead, when I sat in front of my oncologist, she had the same concerned wrinkled forehead, lifted eyebrows and high-pitched, sympathetic, soft voice that my cancer surgeon had five months earlier.

"Linda, we thought your cancer was eradicated. But there was one last step to be sure. We sent the tumors removed during surgery to the lab to analyze. We've learned that one reason cancer returns nine to ten years after surgery in some people is because a few types of tumors spread cancer cells through the blood to the rest of the body using the vein they're growing next to. You have that kind of tumor."

She continued, "There is a 25% chance that your breast cancer cells had already circulated through your system before your surgery. One place where they often metastasize to is the bone. And with bone cancer it can be asymptomatic for nine or more years. When it finally becomes obvious, it's late-stage painful cancer with no known treatment or cure."

"You need chemotherapy to seek out and destroy any possible remaining cancerous cells. Chemotherapy should start soon in order to be effective."

Although I hadn't reacted strongly six months earlier to learning I had cancer for the third time, this chemotherapy news struck me in a completely different way. I've always believed chemo was barbaric and did long-term damage to the body.

Wanting to say, 'no way' and leave, I looked at my oncologist, whom I greatly respected, and said, "Teach me more about why, how and when."

We talked as equals for the next 60 minutes. She respected my questions and understood my resistance.

She is the only reason why, two days later, I acquiesced. I didn't trust the research and science as much as I trusted her.

I called my oncologist's office and said, "Let's start chemo as soon as possible. I want this behind me." Five days later I had my first infusion.

A mere year later, it's my birthday again. Last year I had only just moved to Chico, California, two months earlier and hadn't yet made any real friends. I had celebrated my birthday alone except for two family FaceTime calls. Then, after the visit with my doctor, I spent the rest of my birthday alone, digesting the news of my third cancer diagnosis.

Following my chemo this year in June, I reached out to two new friends and asked them what they were doing on August 31st.

They looked at their calendars and asked, "Why?"

I said, "This date is my birthday, and what I really want is just to go out for dinner with two friends. No gifts. No fancy decorations. Just dinner and conversation."

They asked if they could invite others.

I shrugged and said, "Only if you want to."

Tonight, on my birthday, I walked into the restaurant expecting to join just my two friends. Instead, I was greeted by a long table of 16 people. I was shocked, and they were delighted to surprise me. Many hadn't seen me during the hot month of August when our weather keeps people inside or vacationing elsewhere to escape the 100-plus heat.

When they saw I was no longer bald and had short hair, eyebrows, and eyelashes again, they were doubly excited to see the new re-emerging me.

This party with friends was the best day I've had in over a year. We shared stories, laughed at funny birthday cards, and enjoyed simply celebrating together.

Yes, this year is why we go through chemo—so we can have many more birthdays and fun with people we love.

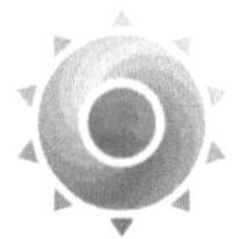

Be Careful What You Wish For—It Might Happen

November 21

AS A SMALL CHILD, like many other little girls, I wanted long, cylindrical curls like those of child movie star Shirley Temple. But when my mother finally acquiesced and gave me a 1950s home permanent, my hair ended up frizzy, looking more like Clarabelle the Clown from the Howdy Doody TV show.

During the 1960s, when other girls were ironing their hair to straighten it and get rid of their curls, my long, middle-of-my-back blonde hair was already straight as a board. No need to flatten it.

Later in the 1970s, when I was working at a YWCA in a mostly black neighborhood in South Philadelphia, the little girls were fascinated with my straight blonde locks. They'd beg me to sit on the steps so they could gather around my head and plait my hair. But when they got to the end of their braids and let go, my hair would promptly unravel and become straight again. They'd laugh and try over and over again, but my hair insisted on returning to its natural, long, straight strands.

All my life I've worked hard to curl my hair, but with the slightest elevation of humidity or just the length of time since it was curled, it would become mostly straight again.

Eventually, I've learned to enjoy my non-curly hair and quit trying to make it different.

While going through chemo I was told by many that after losing one's hair from chemotherapy, it's not unusual for it to grow back curly and often even in a different color. I laughed, sure that my ornery straight hair roots and blonde color genes wouldn't allow that possibility.

When my hair first started to grow back, I was surprised to see that it had turned pure white, and the blonde undertones were gone.

Initially, my half-inch white covering looked like I had deliberately shaved it short. Suddenly, I looked cool to younger generations. When people asked about it, I smiled and said, "I had a million-dollar cut," and then watched their confusion.

As my hair continued to grow, it began to curl into very tight ringlets that refused to be brushed in any direction or styled. I had little corkscrews all over my head. I tried to pull one ringlet straight, but it immediately snapped back into a tight curl as soon as I let go.

Now I no longer look hip as when it was shorter. Instead, I look in a mirror and see an old lady from the 1960s, who went to the beauty parlor to get a perm that gave her tight curls all over her head. I gasp and think, *Oh no! I'm one of those old biddies I promised I'd never become.*

I'd always wanted curly hair. Now I'm getting to experience it full force. Some say that the post-chemo curly hair goes away after several years. Others claim it lasts for life. Predictions once again turn out to be futile as I continue rebuilding my body and look, post-chemo.

If this cancer journey has taught me anything, it's easier to acquiesce to what is than to fight it. More important than obsessing about my hair is reminding myself to continue to grow with empathy towards others and feel gratitude for all who have helped me move through cancer. Being healthy and alive is enough. How I look is secondary or even much further down the list.

I've said that I'll continue to let my hair grow long again, which will take several years, so that I can see how it changes as it grows. Once I've completed this metamorphosis from bald to long hair, I'll decide whether to live with curly locks, returned straight hair, or shave it off and be hip again.

But by then, who knows what hairstyles will be like in two years. I'll just have to decide what I feel like then.

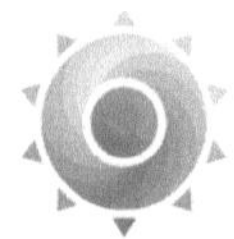

What Do You Call Us?

December 6

A DIFFICULT ASPECT of writing about cancer is knowing what to call those of us experiencing cancer. "Cancer Survivor" is frequently used. But to me this term is like running fingernails down an old chalkboard. I personally loathe this term.

Breast cancer survivor is a name given to people as soon as they are diagnosed with cancer and not after they've survived it. So, on day one, I'm a cancer survivor, continue to be one during treatments, and for the rest of my life.

But I ask, "Isn't everyone in this world a survivor?" Why then do I get to be called a survivor only once I'm diagnosed with cancer? *Survivor before. Survivor now. Survivor afterwards.* So what?

My deeper problem with this term is: *What do we call people like my husband who didn't survive cancer?*

To me, his facing terminal cancer and still wanting to make the most of each precious day as his body continued to decline, makes him more heroic than me, who lived through multiple episodes of cancer. What title do we give those whose lives are ended by cancer? *Are they non-survivors?*

In my writings I needed a different word, so I began by using cancer people. But my daughter, Lindsey, quickly corrected me.

She said, "It's people with cancer."

Wow! How correct. In my writings I keep saying, "I'm more than any disease. Please remember—I'm still Linda." This term, "people with cancer," emphasizes that I am a person, and cancer is only an ancillary part of that whole being.

"Why is language so important?" many ask, frustrated by today's political correctness and renaming. My answer is: "Because it forms how we see, relate, talk, respond, and act towards a person."

Those of us facing cancer and those who love and care about us need ways to see people with cancer as still being whole people. In my writings, I now use the term "people with cancer." And I understand that others with cancer may choose other words including cancer survivor. We don't all share the same preferences, and I honor other persons and organizations word choices.

One of the sayings I'll always remember my mother repeating to me when I got all wound up over multiple causes is: "Choose your battles carefully, because there are so many that could be fought."

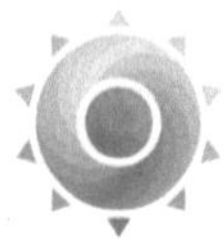

My Body As Clothing

January 4

IT STARTED YESTERDAY after working outside in the garden. I got what I thought looked like several mosquito bites that itched intensely. My reaction was: *What? It's still winter. How did that happen?*

Then the mosquito bites started to multiply all over my backside and looked more like I'd been exposed to poison oak or ivy. Again, I was confused. *These plant leaves aren't even out yet, and I know neither is growing in my yard.*

The bumps continued to spread until the itch was out of control. Finally, I made a call to my dermatologist's office begging for an appointment. The earliest they could squeeze me in was three days later.

I knew my challenge was going to be how to try to be comfortable until I could get an expert's opinion and help. It really was uncomfortable and hard not to scratch. But rubbing one spot only made other places all over my body start to itch, too.

It's sort of like when you ask someone to scratch a hard-to-reach spot on your back and as they do, suddenly more new places suddenly pop up and want attention. You end up begging and directing the scratcher to more and more new places.

I learned during chemo not to say to myself, *I have a headache. I'm dizzy. Oh no, I have a nosebleed.* Instead, I'd say: *My body has a nosebleed*, or *my head aches*. But not: *I AM anything!* I didn't have cancer, but my body or cells had it.

It was a subtle difference but separating my identity from my body allowed me to observe its symptoms from a third-person point of view. And, I'd say to myself, *I'm still this greater "being" separate from my distressed physical body.*

Despite my constant and nearly intolerable itching, I watched it like an outside observer. I noticed that soft clothing next to it felt better. And, since my skin is naturally dry, if I moisturized it with cream, it felt a little better. Exercising, perspiring, and hot showers were negatives. So, I used my chemo detachment skill and immersed myself in writing or preparing for a class I was facilitating. I lost myself in playing Solitaire. I looked for recipes to cook. Anything to engage me and remove focus from my body's discomfort.

When I finally saw my dermatologist, he couldn't identify the rash visually and needed a biopsy. He told me it would take two weeks for the only lab that does this work to send a report. In the meanwhile, a steroid shot might help. I immediately agreed to the shot.

The good news is the shot worked and in three days I was almost back to feeling normal.

But three weeks later, the itching returned full force. The dermatologist said the biopsy report was inconclusive about identifying a cause. He said my breakout and itches might go on indefinitely, if we couldn't more exactly identify it and its source. He could give me a final booster shot of steroids and hope for the best. I immediately agreed to the booster.

He explained that going through chemotherapy changes a body's chemistry, and he had a strong hunch that my skin's reaction was related to my chemo. It may have made me allergic to things I wasn't before. *But allergic to what?*

We talked about the next step of going to an allergist to determine through tests if my skin's reaction was, in fact, an allergy. I asked if the medication I was taking to suppress hormones to keep breast cancer away might be a cause. It was the only real change I could identify.

He pulled out his cell phone, went to an app identifying drug side effects, and typed in my prescription's name. And yep! It showed side effect photos that exactly matched my skin rash.

Amazing how I thought this cancer and chemo journey were over. Here it was sneaking under my walls of protection and saying, *I'm back and not over!*

I stopped taking the prescribed medication and the itchy skin was gone.

I remember being in my twenties, renting a house, and working to turn a backyard of weeds into a lovely garden. Two days later I was covered from head to foot with poison ivy. I tried a variety of minimally effective treatments and went from one doctor to the next looking for a way to handle the itch and distress.

But now, a half century later, having an equally difficult rash and itch, I handled it much differently. Going through 15 weeks of intense physical reaction to chemo followed by another six months of fighting lingering fatigue, I learned how to separate my body from who I really am. This time I didn't become consumed by the symptoms of itching and instead focused on other areas of my life to distract me from its irritation.

It's a skill and perspective I never would have learned without this past year. And I'm grateful I've learned it.

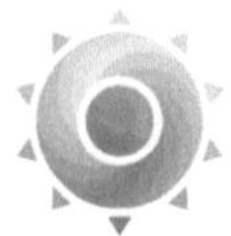

Not the Same Person Who Went Through Chemo

February 14

THIS WEEK, AS I READ through my chemotherapy journal and transferred its entries onto my computer to form this new book, I clearly recognized the feelings and the physical and mental states I had described in my writings over the past year. When I created each, I had not thought of sharing them with others. I wrote each as waves of expressions encompassed me, needing to be released.

I'd grab a pen and my journal that I kept next to my chair where I spent much of my day. I'd begin writing, often feeling like the words were coming not from myself but a third person. Ideas flowed onto paper—raw and unedited. Titles would come, pieces not yet formed into language bumped against my chest, its fragments like a jumbled-up necklace with its strands knotted together. Slowly I'd pull at one loop hoping to untangle the words and reveal what they were trying to say.

When finally expressed, I put down my journal and sat feeling relief. What flowed out no longer constrained me or swirled around my body and brain.

In a quiet mind state that was common after each period of writing, I'd sometimes reread the scribbles I had jotted and formed into sentences, paragraphs, and pages. What I had written felt real, but I'd often marvel at the contents and wonder, *Where did they come from? How had I written anything this expressive and accurate?*

When people ask me if I believe in reincarnation, I always smile and say: "Yes, I've had at least 10 lives in this lifetime alone." That's how I feel when I reread entries written a year ago. They certainly were my experience then, but I no longer feel their hurt, pain, and confusion. I've always said: "Life continually comes together and falls apart. The room created by what's lost gives space for new beginnings."

This chemo year was a challenging period, but it was also a time of real growth. I was forced to face the chemo demon none of us wants to experience. But like all other fears I have dealt with in life—once confronted, the old fear no longer possesses its previous strength to alarm or haunt me.

I hope I never need to go through chemo again, but now I know an inner strength I can use to face similar difficulties in life.

Not only has chemo decreased the possibilities of future cancer, it tore down old walls that no longer served me. I've learned that I don't have to be a superwoman. That it's okay to be less than average. I have huge respect for others going through cancer and am grateful for the advances in medical research that, hopefully, will eradicate or at least deflate cancer's negative effects for so many in the future.

When my writing group said to me this week, "You're brave to share your cancer writings." My thoughts were: *It's not hard to revisit or share. The Linda in these journal writings was the me then who was facing cancer and chemo. I'm a different person now.*

I was sure last year that when my chemo was completed, I'd never want to talk about or revisit that experience. Immediately post-treatment, I hid my cancer journal in my office so I wouldn't have to see it. After chemo I only wanted to focus on enjoying life and building my body back even stronger than before.

Today I feel vibrant again. I wake up excited and ready to explore what's ahead each day.

Now when I share my writings and learn that my words have helped others to understand this difficult journey, I'm grateful they're doing others good. These journal entries helped to heal me. If they assist people in understanding how to support others going through chemotherapy, I'm happy to share them. So, as I reread, edit, and fill in missing pieces, I'm happy with whom I've become post-chemo.

And these writings have helped me clear any remaining baggage from my closets so I can travel through life more lightly.

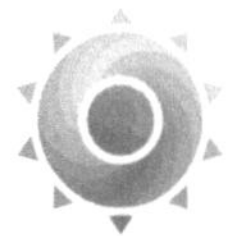

An Anniversary Worth Celebrating

February 15

YEAH! ANOTHER ANNIVERSARY. The kind that's fun to celebrate. A year ago, I started my first chemo treatment. But that's not what I'm celebrating. Why would I celebrate the beginning of such a difficult journey?

Today I'm celebrating my return to great health. I got on the bathroom scales this morning, and I'm once again at my pre-cancer weight. It feels so familiar and terrific.

In January I taught a course titled "Answering What Now in a World of Accelerating Change." One purpose was to help individuals understand how they react to changes they can't control, as well as successfully create others they want in their lives.

I gave the group an exercise, asking them to observe their reaction to change and identify a personal goal they'd like to make happen in their life. Next their assignment was to choose a simple three- to five-minute daily activity that would help them move toward their larger goal. This task was to be so simple that there would be no easy reason why they couldn't do it. At the end of each day, they were to write in a journal one or two sentences about how they did.

The purpose of the exercise was for them to create their own data and observations about how they react to a simple change in their life.

One example I gave them was this: if their goal was to develop an exercise routine, a three- to five-minute activity could be to put on their walking shoes, go outside, and walk around their home once. That's it. Just a small step toward their larger goal.

I told them I was going to participate, too. My goal was to eat healthier and give my body more nutritious foods. My short daily task was to eat a small bag of carrots and celery at four o'clock every afternoon. This is when I get hungry and am tempted to eat too many salted peanuts or, even worse, potato chips. Yep, the thick kind with lots of salt.

What I hoped they might discover is that the hardest part of any new habit is the beginning. Once started, it's easier to escalate the simple exercise—one you had no reason not to do—into something bigger.

And that's what happened with my simple activity. The veggies at four o'clock helped to fill me up so I ate less at dinner time and made healthier choices. That nutritious dinner grew into big salads for lunch and tossing out all my junk food.

Once I had lost my first five pounds, I began eyeing that pair of skinny jeans stuffed into the back of my closet shoved where they couldn't make me feel guilty just looking at them. My success and history of what it takes for me to lose weight gave me the strength to continue eating healthy. I chose the words *I'm eating only foods that are healthy for my post-chemo body,* and not: *I'm on a diet and need to lose weight.* The healthy food goal was less laden with old history. And I did want my body to be strong again.

This morning, I got on my scales, weighed myself, and marked the results on my wall calendar. My body had finally shed its last pounds gained during my cancer journey. And, I'm wearing my skinny jeans.

During the regularly scheduled three-month follow-up appointment with my oncologist last month, I asked for a referral to a doctor who could help me with my arthritis. I knew a side effect of the hormone-suppressive medicine I need to take for five to ten more years can cause osteoporosis and arthritis. I had found that several of my fingers were swollen, and I couldn't sleep the whole night without awakening several times with hip pain and needing to turn over to the other side. Also, when working in the garden or with any activity where I needed to bend over, my back would hurt for the next several days.

I cringe when people talk about how a new diet solved all their health issues. I avoid listening to cure-all testimonials, having tried to follow too many without the same miraculous results advertised.

But several days ago, I noticed how strong my body has become again. I feel 10 years younger. The aging effects that I felt during chemo when I wrote about knowing what it's like to be old have dissolved.

My hands feel normal, and when I wear my favorite rings, many are loose on my hands again. I'm sleeping deeply through the night and never awaken with hip pain. I've dug up several large garden beds, replanting the crowded iris, cannas, and lilies. The next day my back is fine, and I can continue my gardening.

My body is getting younger and healthier again.

Is it my new healthy diet? Is it because my body has recovered from chemo? Is it because I've finally been able to be socially active and made so many new friends? Is it because my business is picking up, and I'm being asked to speak again and sell my first book? Is it because I'm crossing off items on my endless to-do lists that had only grown longer last year when I was unable to check off items?

Probably all of the above was responsible for why I finally feel like myself again and am filled with excitement about new things I want to accomplish.

My cancer and chemo journey greatly disrupted my life during the last 12 months. But for me, there is a return to feeling not only like myself, but like an even better version of me. I'm privileged to have had great medical, spiritual, and personal support from the medical community, family, neighbors, and friends.

There is no longer a need to hide my cancer writings. They reflect the journey I experienced. But now it's time to focus on my identity not as a former person with cancer, but as the complete person I am with so many accumulated experiences. Cancer merges into that collective whole and no longer is more important than the many other experiences—both good and bad—that have defined and made me who I am today.

As with all fears that we've carried and then faced, chemo will never again have the ability to haunt me. I know it firsthand. It's a bear, but it's helped make me a more compassionate person. One that's easier for me to live with and enjoy.

I embrace this familiar feeling of health and smile with great gratitude that it's time to ask once again, *What Now?* And smile as I carve out my next chapter, or should I say another reincarnation of this lifetime?

PART 2:

Etiquette—What to Say & Not Say or Do

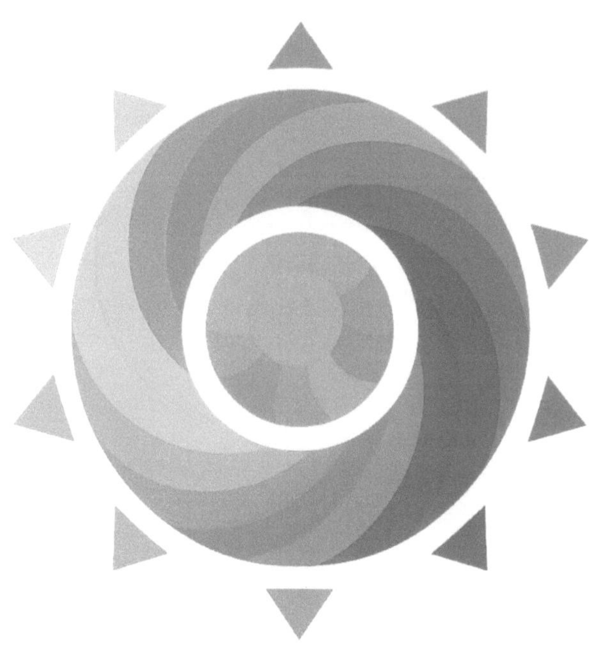

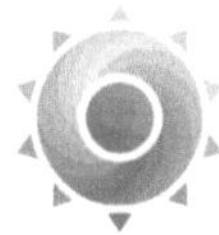

Basic Cancer Etiquette

ETIQUETTE GUIDELINES have been created to help us understand how to best act in social situations. So why not similarly use suggested cancer etiquette to help us know how to behave and communicate with a person experiencing cancer and its challenging treatments?

We all realize that there are a multitude of social etiquette practices and that they don't universally apply to all situations. So, use the ones listed in this section as guidelines for appropriate behavior.

Whenever I speak about my experiences as both a caregiver for my husband with advanced cancer as well as multiple experiences with my own cancer, the most often asked questions are: "How should I act?" "What should I say/not say to a person with cancer and undergoing its treatments?"

The challenge of writing any etiquette guidelines is that there is great variation in both social situations and preferences of people with cancer. There is an even wider range of cancer types, diagnoses, and treatment plans.

While experiencing cancer and its difficult treatments, I sometimes felt normal and wanted to have conversations about other shared interests, rather than discuss my ongoing health situation.

But other days, I was overwhelmed by symptoms and emotions and needed support. On these days I wanted someone to listen and understand my cancer journey. So, it's impossible to give blanket advice that fits all situations and all individuals. Taking each day as it comes is a mantra for many experiencing serious illnesses and should be adopted by friends, family, and other supporters as well. What works and is appropriate today may need to be changed and revised tomorrow.

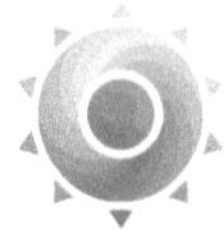

Etiquette Guidance

THE FOLLOWING GUIDANCE is intended to give generalized awareness about what it feels like to be on the receiving side of cancer conversations and interactions so that you can be more sensitive and choose appropriate communications and actions.

Listening Is Your Greatest Asset

Most of us are overly concerned about what to say or not say in conversations with people with cancer. Listening to the person and picking up clues from their behavior is more valuable than anything we have to say or offer them.

Instead of wondering, "What should I say or do?" focus on what the individual with cancer is showing you nonverbally. Also, listen not only to what they're saying, but more importantly how they're delivering it. Don't worry if you end up sharing a moment of silence together. This is often more meaningful than words, especially if your demeanor is calm.

Guideline 1: Be a good listener.

- This will be your greatest guide for what to say or not say. Allow them to tell or not tell their story in their own way.
- While listening, feel free to ask questions to clarify what they've expressed, but don't jump in with your own stories or offer advice.

Guideline 2: Respect a person's privacy about their health and treatments.

- Let them bring up what they're ready to share, when the time is right for them. They may feel uncomfortable giving details or know little themselves at that time.
- They may just need a break from talking about their health on a day(s) when it can feel all-consuming.

Guideline 3: Don't feel a need to fill in silent spaces in conversations.

- Feel free to simply share moments of quiet within the conversation wherever they naturally fall.
- For some people, continual conversation can be exhausting. Silence won't be awkward for you if you can relax and be present in the current shared moment.

Guideline 4: Remember we all are more than any health issue.

- Normal everyday conversation is welcomed on most days. We are more than just our disease and treatments.
- Talk about their interests, provide updates on shared activities, friends, and groups.
- Bring a hobby or activity to visits to do together without much talking.

Respect Boundaries & Privacy

Each person with cancer has to decide how much privacy they need, and what are their boundaries in sharing with others about their cancer and treatments.

Guideline 5: If they don't tell you about their cancer, please don't be offended.

- One of the important decisions any person with cancer makes is when and whom they choose to tell. And don't be surprised if the person decides to limit their story to a few people.
- A problem with telling many people about your cancer is that, as soon as most learn about it, they treat you differently and/or ask for constant updates.
- This updating is exhausting for both the person with cancer and caregivers if they have them. A trip anywhere can mean many repetitive conversations about treatments

and progress. This becomes even harder if the prognosis is not good, or a treatment isn't working.

- And I repeat: "We all need time away from our cancer, and we're more than just a disease."

Guideline 6: Don't tell others about a person's cancer unless they've asked you to be their spokesperson.

- A person with cancer or their caregiver may ask you to keep their family, friends, or acquaintances updated with specific information.
- But watch out for the gossip and misinformation that can come from repeated sharing or when people fill in the blanks with their own thoughts.

Guideline 7: Don't assume the person with cancer knows a lot about the specifics of their cancer.

- Asking for many details about their cancer or treatments may work against their personal way of dealing with cancer and make them uncomfortable.
- Every person with cancer chooses their own method for coping.
- Some only want to know enough to make informed decisions about their treatments. Then they cope by focusing as much as they can on everything else in their lives.
- Others want to know every factor about their cancer including detailed descriptions, meaning of vocabulary,

research statistics, treatment options/choices, and what to expect with each decision and development. For this group, learning is a way of regaining control of their life.

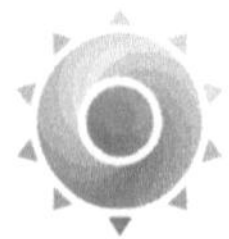

Conversations Guidelines

THE DIFFICULTY WE ALL FACE in deciding what to say to a person facing cancer, and any other life-threatening circumstance, is that there is no one-size-fits-all answer about what to say or even do. But when I talk to others who are experiencing cancer, we share many of the same preferences. In this section, we'll examine some general options for etiquette focusing on our conversations. But please, use your own common sense to fit your specific interactions.

Basic Communications for All Situations

Most of the time the following Guidelines 8-16 will universally apply to all of your communications with people with cancer whether you're in a public setting or in a private one.

Guideline 8: Continue to engage with the person, even if you fear saying the wrong thing.

- If you are a friend, family member, or colleague—keep that relationship by continuing to provide the support you offered before an illness. The individual may have different needs after diagnosis, but they will continue to need a community that helps them feel normal. Just be yourself and let them be themselves as well.

Guideline 9: Don't share your own cancer experiences and thoughts unless specifically asked.

- It's normal for all of us when we hear or read anything new to immediately apply it to what we already know or have experienced. So, when we hear that the person we are talking to has been diagnosed with cancer, we are reminded of our own experiences with cancer, what we've read or learned, and memories of people we know who had cancer. Our immediate natural inclination is to immediately share the details of our cancer experiences with the person we're talking to, but don't.
- These are *your* stories. A person going through cancer shouldn't have to listen to or be sympathetic about other people's experiences or hear about others who may have been diagnosed with something completely different or faced worse or better outcomes. Diagnoses and treatments are unique, and your story or information likely has little relevance to theirs.

- However, if the person with cancer asks for more details about your experiences, tips on what helped with your nausea during treatment or what foods still tasted good and were easy to digest may be helpful to them. Although these anecdotes are still personal, tips like these may help someone new to a diagnosis or treatment. But again, only share if first asked for information.

Guideline 10: Even if you think you know a lot about cancer, don't offer cancer advice.

- The most I ever say to a person with cancer is, "Are you happy with the way your medical professionals are helping you with your cancer?"
- If they reply yes, then I express gratitude that they have support they trust.
- But if they say no, I might ask if they'd like help learning about alternative resources.

Guideline 11: Be careful not to offer unsolicited medical advice or question someone's medical decisions.

- During my husband's cancer I heard endless advice about treatments that had helped someone's relative or how an alternative medical treatment not used by our established medical doctors had worked miracles.
- People emailed me articles about magical cures or recent stories in the news. I was gifted books on cancer to read to him and given vitamins and pills he should take.

- I was surprised how insistent some people could be that we had to try their remedy or see their doctor. It's hard enough facing cancer without defending your medical decisions to others.
- Deciding not to receive certain treatments is also a personal choice we need to respect.

Guideline 12: When learning about their condition, don't say: "I know how you feel."

- My internal reaction to such statements would have been, *No, you don't.*
- Everyone's experience with cancer is unique.
- There are too many kinds of cancer, stages of development, and treatment options for our experiences to be parallel. And each of us processes difficulties differently.

Guideline 13: Don't search for positives by saying, "At least it's not" a disease or condition you think is worse.

- There is no need to search for benefits like: "At least you'll get more time away from the office." Or, "Now you'll have more time to spend with your family."
- You can say that you wished it hadn't happened or that it's a difficult thing they're dealing with. That may feel truer than false platitudes to a person who is still coming to terms with a diagnosis.

Guideline 14: Never say: "Everything happens for a reason."

- This is another tired expression that can be unintentionally hurtful. Similarly, attributing causes (like smoking) to cancer may make you feel better if you're a non-smoker, but it may be both medically incorrect and certainly unhelpful to the individual facing a difficult diagnosis.

Guideline 15: Don't tell people to "be strong" or say, "You'll get through it."

- Some days, we don't feel strong. Some days, making it through a hard day is enough.
- It's okay for people with cancer to be weak, to have bad days, and to feel anger or sadness at the unexpected changes in their lives.
- Regardless of how strong a person has been before cancer—the reality is that some won't make it through.

Guideline 16: Don't expect the person with cancer to educate you about the basics of cancer.

- It is your job to learn some of the basic terminology so that you can be supportive.
- In cancer support groups this is one of the biggest complaints about dealing with others. We feel that we have to explain repeatedly a lot of the *basics about cancer* to other people.

- After talking to a person with cancer, look up the words you don't understand. Go to websites of cancer organizations and medical education platforms to learn more. Make sure you understand the medical definition of cancer, the different stages of cancer and their significance in diagnosis. Learn common words like metastasis, chemotherapy, malignant, benign, sarcoma, remission, cancer staging, and palliative care.

Communications at Public Gatherings

Now let's explore conversations in public settings. When you meet a person going through cancer, it's important to realize that anyone new may drop in on what you assumed was a private conversation.

Also, when a person with cancer is out in public, they may not want to think or be reminded about their cancer. They are there to be with others.

The following Guidelines 17-20 are suggested points about appropriate ways to talk with people with cancer in public situations.

Guideline 17: Don't start your conversation with "How are you?"

- It is natural to greet others this way and normally we don't expect an answer, and most of us slough off a real or detailed response. But when something isn't right in our life, it's harder to pretend that all is well. It often feels like a lie, to casually ignore the question.

- When someone who is going through cancer steps out in public, they may not want to discuss their health or explain details of their treatment to others. A commonly used greeting such as "How are you?" may trigger thoughts about their cancer and leave them struggling with how to truthfully respond when the answer isn't "fine."
- When I chose to be out in the world, I didn't want to check in with my feelings, talk about my cancer or, most importantly, fabricate a polite lie to cover up a difficult response to how I was. I just wanted to be Linda.

Guidelines 18: Do greet them by saying: "It's so nice to see you." Or, "I've missed you."

- Or, say anything you would have said to them before they had cancer that doesn't require them to report on their own health.

Guideline 19: At social gatherings, include them in normal conversation about the event.

- Being treated normally is such a relief.
- If they've missed recent gatherings, feel free to update them about significant or funny happenings, just as you would any other person who had been absent.

Guideline 20: Don't approach strangers in public settings to talk about their presumed cancer.

- I discussed the problems I faced with strangers approaching me in public about my cancer in Part 1 of this book in the journal entry titled "No Longer Invisible."

- Attending a recent concert, I saw a woman wearing a popular cancer cap with no hair sticking out beneath it anywhere. My heart immediately engaged, and my first response was to go over to her and offer encouragement about her presumed chemotherapy. But I stopped myself. I remembered what I had written in my journal about when I was out in public and how much I needed to forget about my own cancer and enjoy a normal aspect of my life. And how, when well-meaning people came up to me to share encouraging words about my hair growing back or the temporary nature of my treatment, my escape from cancer-life immediately incinerated.

  So, I held back, even though I longed to reach out to her, and gave her the privacy she deserved. It's amazing when the roles switch how easy it is to forget what we've initially experienced, learned, and then forgotten.

- A friend of mine had badly damaged hair so she asked her hair stylist to give her a very short haircut. Being in good health, she was surprised by the number of women who approached to give her well-meaning encouragement about facing cancer. When observing a stranger we suspect has cancer, remember that our assumptions may be wrong. But even if they aren't, they are definitely irrelevant, and we shouldn't act on them.

Communications with Caregivers and Family Members

When meeting, talking, or emailing caregivers or family members, the following applies.

Guideline 21: Don't assume that caregivers and family want to give updates or talk about their family member.

- Not everyone close to a person with cancer feels comfortable giving updates about them. Don't be surprised if when you ask you get a reply like: "I don't feel comfortable talking about Chris." Or "I'm letting Jose talk for himself."

Guideline 22: Even if the person has offered updates in the past, never start your conversation with them by asking about the person with cancer.

- Always start by talking normally about things you've discussed in the past before asking how they and the person with cancer is doing.

Social Media Communications

For many of us, using social media is a way to stay up to date on family, friends, and social contacts. It's important to remember that social media posts stay around indefinitely and are often reposted to others.

This is an area where etiquette is especially needed. Some people going through cancer are very public about their condition and readily welcome support on social media from not only those they know, but also others as well. However, never assume they want their cancer publicly shared on any social media or in other news-distribution methods.

Guidelines 23: If the person with cancer hasn't posted about their condition online, don't mention it in any of your posts or comments.

- As soon as one friend mentioned in a private comment to me on social media that I was going through chemotherapy, suddenly ads about cancer started popping up on my social media pages and even on other browser ones. I was bombarded for weeks with unwanted reminders of my cancer. Her comment had changed my invisible profile, and I felt powerless to correct it.

Guidelines 24: Don't recirculate anyone's personal posts about cancer unless they have given you permission or specifically asked you to do so.

Written Communications

Emails, cards, letters, messaging, and other forms of written communications have several additional etiquette guidelines.

Guideline 25: Cards with personal notes are welcome because they can be opened and read as the recipient has energy and time.

- Receiving physical cards can be used as decorations and helps remind the person that they are not forgotten.
- Don't send a "Get Well" greeting card to a person who is facing a long-term healing process and/or a terminal diagnosis. These cards were meant for people with a short-term curable health problem.
- Do send "thinking of you" cards. This is a more appropriate and meaningful gesture to a person when getting well may not be in the probable future.
- Do add your own note to any card. This personalizes the card and conveys your own communication with them.

Guideline 26: Make sure you know the electronic habits of the person you're sending communications to.

- Unfortunately, not everyone has set up "do not disturb" times on their electronics. Make sure the times you're sending messages won't disturb them.
- Your message may not be seen if the person isn't feeling able to continue to use former styles of communications or regularly check for updates.

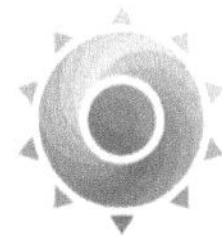

Visit Guidelines

THE FOLLOWING ADVICE IS SPECIFIC to when you visit someone with cancer while they remain in their own home or are being treated in a hospital or care facility.

Home Visits

Guideline 27: Always make sure a home visit is desired and scheduled at the best time for the person with cancer.

- Then, before showing up, reconfirm shortly before the visit (an hour or two is best) to make sure that they still feel up to a visit.

  I had a hard time knowing how I'd feel each day during chemotherapy. So, it was nice when a person checked in to see if our scheduled visit was still appropriate or needed rescheduling.

Guideline 28: Keep visits short.

- When people visited my husband after his health had declined severely, he often suddenly perked up and put on a much cheerier front when visitors arrived. And despite his poor health, he enjoyed the time spent with them. But after long visits, he'd come crashing down as soon as they left, having spent too much valuable energy talking and interacting. The price he paid for an overly long visit was too expensive.
- If a person has a caregiver, ask about the appropriate length for your visit when you arrive. And always leave, if possible, while the individual you're visiting is still feeling relaxed and happy.

Guideline 29: Realize even simple conversations can be exhausting.

- One reason I didn't invite friends to visit when I wasn't feeling well was because I felt an obligation to entertain them. Instead, what I needed was shared, easy time with my company.
- I wish I could have said, "Come over but bring something to do to amuse yourself like something to read or watch on your phone, so I won't need to talk the whole time."

Hospital or Care Facility Visits

Naturally, all the etiquette suggestions about home visits apply to hospital and care facilities—with a few extras.

Guideline 30: Make sure first to check with any caregiver or family members about whether a visit is desirable, and if so, what's the best timing.

- Hospitals and care facilities can be exhausting experiences with so many medical personnel continuously entering and exiting the person's room.
- Quiet times may be needed for sleep and rest.

Guideline 31: Respect the privacy of the patient without being asked.

- Quietly exit the room when a medical person enters to talk about their health or to do any medical procedure or personal-care activity.

Guideline 32: Don't bring gifts that take up valuable shelf space in the patient's room.

- Many facilities don't provide a place to set flowers and gifts. And happy balloons can get tangled up with medical equipment.
- I remember how difficult it was each time my husband was discharged from a hospital to transport him, all his own personal stuff, and the gifts brought by visitors to the car. It was an overwhelming task. As a caregiver all I wanted to do was make sure he was safe and comfortable during the journey home.

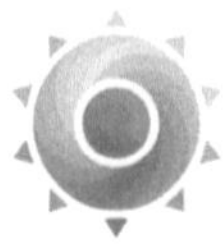

The Prayer Dilemma Etiquette

AS WE WERE DRIVING home from an event, a friend of mine told me that her husband was just diagnosed with Stage 4 cancer. I listened as she went into greater details. As she talked, I followed my number one rule—listen to the person and don't interrupt with your own stories or give advice before asked.

The diagnosis was so recent that they were still waiting for more test results, considering treatment options, and determining what kind of surgery—if any—is suggested.

I asked how she was handling this news and listened to her responses. She revealed that exploratory surgery, scheduled for about two weeks out, would reveal more about his cancer. The exact date hadn't been set yet. I understood well the challenges of scheduling a surgery date, as it involves not only the surgeon's calendar but also operating room availability and hospital staffing.

I asked what kind of support she needed while she waited. Her response was as I had anticipated—she didn't know. Since I see her at a weekly event, I knew I'd hear more in the upcoming weeks.

But wanting to offer something immediately, I made a huge error and said, "I'll pray for his health and well-being."

After a long silence she responded, "I'm uncomfortable with the word 'pray.' My husband is an atheist. Knowing that people are praying for him would be an invasion of his personal beliefs."

I silently reprimanded myself. I had made an assumption that broke rules of etiquette. In social situations, unsolicited personal religious beliefs should never be offered.

I paused, realizing she was right. My goal was to offer her and her husband support, and what I had just said caused her more stress. I failed in my desire to be supportive.

For those of us who believe in the power of sending healing thoughts, prayers, or any other kind of helpful energy, we need to be conscious of the beliefs of the person we're talking to before verbally offering this kind of unrequested support. The same applies to letters or cards that offer prayers or other religious messages. We need to ask ourselves whether they will be welcomed by the recipient.

I wish I had phrased my offer as a question rather than as a direct statement. I could have said, "Would you and your husband welcome prayers or healing thoughts?" Her answer would have given me boundaries for what she would consider supportive.

When Bill was first diagnosed with terminal cancer, we both were overwhelmed by the unexpected news. Hearing people express love and offer support as needed was all we could process at that time.

What I especially didn't need in those early days was having to manage other people's panic and emotions as they shared their thoughts about what this diagnosis meant for me and my family. Outsiders who have just heard about someone's diagnosis of cancer need time to process the news themselves—but it's not the job of the caregiver or person with cancer to support them through that process.

Some friends, family members, and would-be supporters had to be gently pushed out of our lives because they made the situation harder rather than more bearable. I kept a short list of people my husband didn't want to talk to—those who were too needy and emotionally draining for him.

Our goal should be to support the individual affected by a cancer diagnosis. And we need to be careful that the timing and nature of our offers for help are appropriate and welcome. In this way we can truly support them, rather than making an already difficult time even more challenging.

PART 3:
50+ Support Ideas

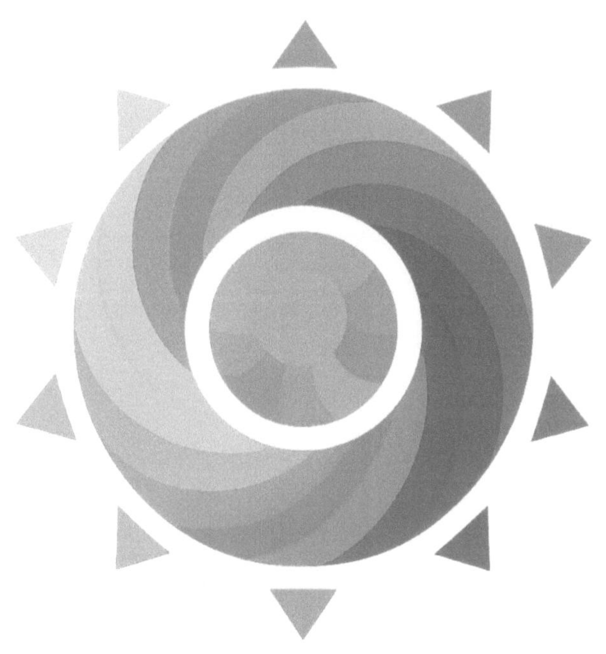

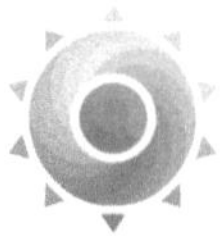

Support Ideas Introduction

IT'S HUMAN NATURE TO WANT to help others facing difficult times, which often mirror our own worst fears. When hearing unsettling news, it's normal to think that this could be me or someone I deeply care about.

Just because a person is diagnosed with some form of cancer doesn't mean they immediately or automatically need a lot of volunteer support to assist them with a wide variety of daily tasks. There are so many different types of cancer and, when diagnosed early in beginning stages, treatments may not significantly impact their life.

This section is intended to help you understand how to support those whose health is compromised by cancer and some of its more challenging treatments. These ideas are also relevant for anyone wanting to assist other people experiencing difficult times regardless of their health circumstances or personal challenges.

Historically, the most common way of helping people has been by bringing unsolicited food and flowers. But there are many other ways to be useful.

First, reflect on all the daily, weekly, and monthly tasks you do for yourself, your home, vehicles, children, and pets. The person with cancer will have similar needs and tasks and may welcome your assistance.

Second, think about your talents, expertise, gifts, or activities that you enjoy. Is it organizing things, coordinating resources, technology, baking, gardening, pets, children, organizing people, shopping, driving places? These are possible areas where someone whose life has been made more difficult by cancer may appreciate help.

The list of support ideas in this section is not meant to be exhaustive. Rather, use these suggestions to stimulate ones of your own.

The Difficulty of General "Anything" Offers

The most common offer is, "Let me know what I can do to help?" But these blanket offers put the responsibility on the person facing cancer to initiate a help request. And often when assistance is needed, it can be very specific. Like: "I need a ride next Tuesday morning at 8:30 a.m. to a two-hour appointment 20 miles away."

When the person with cancer calls someone who offered unspecified help, they face the possibility that the person already is busy or may not be interested in supporting in that specific way. It's also awkward for both if the person asked can't help that day or that way.

As I mentioned in Part 1 of this book, I had plenty of initial offers of assistance, but I was overwhelmed with my treatment preparation, and I've never been good at asking for help. Weeks after the offers were made, I was weaker and needed some support. But I was no longer sure who had made what offer and if the person I wanted to ask would still be willing and available to help me. Most of all, I didn't want to be a burden to others.

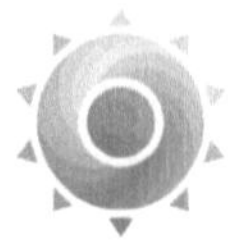

Specific 50+ Support Ideas

TIME AND ENERGY CAN BECOME precious commodities for cancer patients and their caregivers. The following are fifty specific ideas about how to support those whose lives are consumed by managing their health and/or facing difficult transitions.

When you make an offer of support, describe how you might be able to help, but don't be offended if the person doesn't take you up on your suggestion immediately. They may initially be inundated with offers—to bring meals, provide rides, visit—and not able to determine when or if they'll need and want them.

If you're still available to provide support over time, continue to check back in about their needs and restate some specific ways you'd like to help out.

Support Network Coordination

Offers can come from so many sources—family, friends, social groups, neighbors, work/business groups. This network coordination section suggests ways to volunteer to organize support efforts for a specific group.

1 **Communications support person for specific group**: ask if they'd like you to be the person to interface with a specific group to share health updates and organize support offers.

- The emotional drain of re-explaining medical and personal information is significant, but be sure to confirm how much the individual wants to share with others in different social, business, or family circles before providing any information.
- Giving updates and answering questions on behalf of the person with cancer gives them and their caregivers more time to recover from treatments.

2 **Online support coordination**: there are many websites on the internet that offer ways to organize and coordinate volunteer support. Some sites provide a calendar for scheduling meals or rides for appointments, and others present ways to share more detailed information about an individual's health. With their approval, set-up, manage, and coordinate one of these services on their behalf, based on their ever-changing needs.

- The American Cancer Society is one place to look for suggested and vetted websites to help individuals organize online volunteer support for people with cancer.
- Do an online search with wording like "website to coordinate volunteer support for people with cancer" to find other possible sites.

Home Management

Think of all the things you routinely do around your home. Then volunteer to do some of these same household tasks.

3 **House cleaning**: this service can be one you offer to do yourself or give a gift certificate for a cleaning service to come and clean for them. Remember that harsh chemicals may be harmful to those with difficult breathing or sensitive skin.

4 **Bed making and changing**: can be a daunting task for someone with limited mobility, or for a caregiver to do on their own. Making a bed with fresh sheets and washing towels and linens helps them stay healthier and happier during treatments.

5 **Window washing**: often a great gift to someone who is house bound and must spend a lot of time inside. Windows may be one of their bridges to the outside world. Even washing a single window next to a favorite chair or bed can be enough to bring joy.

6 **Clothes**: washing, mending, and dry cleaning are weekly tasks we all need to do. Doing these chores for a person with cancer creates an opportunity to spend time with them while the washer and dryer are running.

7 **Mail sorting**: piles can accumulate quickly and feel overwhelming when we worry that important information and bills may become buried under junk mail. Offer to identify items to be tossed, bills to be paid or filed, and personal mail or cards to be opened.

8 **Outside flower basket or bird feeder**: hanging one outside a window where the person spends a lot of time can provide visual interest for someone experiencing more time at home.

9 **Yard work, gardening, outdoor maintenance**: when physical and mental energy is diverted to medical care, outdoor chores can be the first to fall behind. Offer specific help based on your abilities and their needs—from pulling weeds, to tending flowers, to completing handy person tasks.

10 **Garbage/recycling day support**: most people have specific days for their trash and recycling pickups. Find out by what method and on which days trash is collected. Then coordinate help if needed. This is a great way for neighbors to help since they are already nearby and are doing the same tasks for themselves.

11 **Mail pick-ups**: if they have a mailbox out on the road or on the street, picking up and delivering mail to their door is a simple task for neighbors, but a real gift on difficult days.

12 **Post Office, UPS, or other mailing center offers**: if you're heading to one, check to see if the person you're helping has any drop offs or items needing postage.

- In this day of online ordering, a reality is returns of items that we don't want. But standing in line to make a return can be a chore.
- Especially remember this offer around gift-giving holidays if they celebrate any. They may need help wrapping, packing, and sending items.

Car or Vehicle

13 **Vehicle washing and cleaning**: who doesn't enjoy getting into a freshly cleaned car, van, or truck? This simple gesture can offer a special lift. Do the work yourself or take it to a car wash or car-detailing service.

14 **Inspections, license renewals, and oil changes**: ask when they need to have their car inspected, oil changed, tires rotated, or other maintenance performed. Things like this often get missed or forgotten when your brain isn't working at full capacity due to medication, treatments and/or lack of energy.

- I drove my car with the message "maintenance required" staring at me from my dashboard during the six months of post-surgery and chemo because I didn't have the energy to take my car to the dealership and wait while the maintenance department checked it out. It turned out to simply be a 25,000-mile routine checkup, but it caused me a lot of anxiety because I didn't know what the issue was and every time I got in the car, the message reappeared.

Food

Most people think immediately about bringing food to a person in a time of need. But since this continuous need for help with food and meals may expand across longer periods of time, also consider the following suggestions.

15 **Prepared food**: the best kinds are those that can be delivered in non-returnable, microwavable safe containers that can be reheated. I've heard of friends who had three large lasagna pans arrive around the same time from different people. Make sure the meals are coordinated and needed.

- Appetites can change when recovering or while receiving different treatments, so check to be sure the meals/food sound appetizing to the individual, in addition to meeting their food preferences and dietary requirements.
- Soft, easy-to-swallow foods may be necessary for people with advanced or severe illnesses when it sometimes becomes difficult to chew and swallow. Frozen Italian Ices were my husband's favorites, but he

needed non-acidic flavors like cherry or watermelon instead of lemon or lime.

16 **Grocery home-delivery gift certificates**: are a great way to offer food. It allows the recipient to select what they need and then have it delivered to their home.

- Certificates are great because they can be used any time. Often during extended periods where support is needed, this kind of gift can be extremely appreciated.
- It's also perfect for caregivers who don't know how to cook, lack time to shop, or supporters who live far away.
- Many food stores offer their own food shopping and delivery services. Check to see if the person uses one of these or would like to learn how to use them.

17 **Website foods**: that can be ordered and sent directly allow the person to both order the food and then eat it when needed.

18 **Grocery shop**: for them by creating a list with the person and then picking up the specific items they need. Often people also need non-food items like paper towels, toilet paper, hand lotion, etc., so remember to ask them which of these items they may need.

Medical Information Organization

19 **Medical research:** at the beginning of being diagnosed, some people need help learning more about their

disease and options. If you enjoy research, ask if they'd like your help finding information and options.

20 **Medical documents sorting and filing**: It's amazing how many medical-related information sheets, brochures, and items are collected from different medical providers. Add to this their daily mail (email or snail mail) delivering medical and insurance bills/statements. If you have a talent for sorting these documents and organizing them, this can be greatly appreciated.

Medications Support

21 **Drugstore shopping**: if you're headed to a drug store, check and see if you can pick up any special supplies or prescriptions for them.

22 **Medication runs**: often as a person leaves the hospital, they may receive new prescriptions that need to be filled. Offer to pick these up as soon as they are called in by the doctor or hospital. Waiting for home delivery by the pharmacy often takes too long.

23 **Medications organization**: often it gets hard to organize all the medication bottles and packages and remember when to take each. The following ideas may help organize these medications:

- **Help label and organize medications** into day-of-the-week pill containers sorting them by timing and frequency of each medication. Provide a list of easy-to-read instructions.

- **For a complex list make a master list of medications** by reading all the fine print on their behalf and noting on the list amounts to be taken, time of day, whether they are required or optional, and taken with/without food. Setting up alarms using timers for frequent doses may help.

Support During Visits

As discussed earlier, people often feel obliged to entertain their visitors and put on a brave front. Here are a few reminders to keep in mind when you're the one visiting.

24 **Short visits**: living with cancer or many other diseases means managing energy and not just time. Often, people won't show you their true limitations, and visits can be very tiring. Leave while the person is still appreciating your visit.

25 **Share space instead of conversation**: in more advanced stages of cancer and treatments, when energy may be limited, even simple talking can become a chore. So, prepare to sit and enjoy sharing the same space with the person you're visiting without demanding ongoing conversation.

- When you talk to a person unable to be conversational, tune down your own energy, speak more slowly, and use fewer words.

- I'm a knitter, and I often take my knitting when I visit someone. It allows them to relax and even sleep, knowing that I don't need to be entertained.

26 **Watch TV or a movie together or listen to music**: these less demanding activities can replace conversations and allow the person to nap if they need the rest.

27 **Read to the person**: is another excellent activity that allows them to relax, shut their eyes, and only listen. I was so tired some days that reading for myself took too much effort. But I had a list of reading materials I would have loved someone to read to me. So, ask if there is anything they'd like you to read to them.

28 **Read their cards or emails they've received to them**: this can be most welcome. When I saw a long personal message on days when my strength was low, I often set it aside to be read at another time.

Communications-Written & Online

29 **Cards with personal notes**: are welcome because they can be opened and read as the recipient has energy and time. Often the cards can also be used as decorations.

- But remember as I mentioned in the Etiquette Section, do not send a "Get Well" greeting card to a person who is facing a long-term healing process or a terminal diagnosis. These cards are best for people with a short-term, curable health problem. When "getting well" isn't a probable future, greeting cards with a more personal written message are ideal.

30 **Social media**: writing short notes on social media is a common way to keep in touch with friends. But don't use social media unless you've communicated this way with the person in the past. And make sure you only respond to them personally, not as a "reply all," unless they've first posted something inviting comments from everyone.

- I chose not to use social media to share that I had cancer again. Social media posts stay forever. I didn't want people I'd meet in the future or potential clients/ employers to find out about my cancer for an infinite time in the future.

Transportation to Appointments

31 **Transportation needs identification**: find out if the person needs transportation to medical appointments, tests, and treatments.

- Check out websites or apps that offer calendars that can be created and accessed with the appropriate code to sign up online for transportation to medical visits.
- Some cancer organizations and medical institutions offer free transportation. Offer to research these possibilities for the person with cancer and fill out applications, if needed to use them.

32 **Handicapped-parking pass procurement & usage**: this pass is especially appreciated when going to appointments. Make sure to take one, if available, with you so that you can park close to entrances. If the person with cancer doesn't have one, offer to contact their physician's office to initiate the process for them receiving one.

Outside Home Entertainment

For those undergoing treatment, leaving home can be a chore reserved only for medical visits. But if they are interested in getting outside, offer to take them out on short, low-impact activities. Be prepared, however, to cancel or change plans at the last minute, based on their energy and health.

33 **Short recreational drives**: a new favorite activity may simply be a ride around their area so they can see the spring flowers, fall leaves, or holiday lights.

34 **Favorite restaurant**: reserve an easy-access table in advance for a meal out. Be prepared to take leftovers home and leave early if the individual gets tired.

35 **Movie or concert**: some people may want company for a movie or concert to have a break from being at home. Caregivers may appreciate the time to recuperate for themselves as well. Try going to movies at off-hours or to matinees with fewer crowds, less overwhelming noise, and less exposure to others for those with compromised immune systems.

Technology Support

Encourage assistance from tech-savvy friends and family to help the person keep up with daily mobile devices and computer tasks that can seem overwhelming even when in good health.

36 **Email assistance**: reading and responding to emails and other correspondence.

- Add organizational filters to sort types of messages or unsubscribe from unwanted newsletters or promotional emails.

37 **Online health system support**: help with login information or filling out health information prior to doctors' visits.

- Most medical offices and testing centers have their own apps and websites, resulting in many logins to keep organized and duplicated information to be filled in.

38 **Computer accessibility improvements**: make things like changing the size of text on the screen or creating shortcuts to sign in to email or social media easier.

39 **Computer maintenance**: if you are confident in your technology abilities offer to upgrade systems, troubleshoot problems, and keep security up-to-date.

40 **Streaming service set up**: help subscribe for easier entertainment on TV, computer, or mobile device.

Financial Assistance—Sorting & Applications

For some individuals who are experiencing cancer and its treatments, managing finances can be overwhelming. This is made especially taxing by foggy thinking from medications and chemotherapy.

If you have financial skills and/or understand insurance, payments or how to apply for financial assistance, your help could be invaluable to a person juggling many medical bills.

41 **Medical bills sorting:** to organize and identify ones to be paid.

- Separate bills sent by different doctors, hospitals, labs, and testing centers.
- Even when a person has health insurance, it can be a difficult task tracking what bills are owed after health insurance payments are received and required deductions are met.

42 **Financial support applications assistance**: from medical institutions if needed for financial relief.

Family Support & Caregivers Relief

43 **Babysitting or other family support**: can include supporting children of all ages living with them.

- Get them out of the house for a fun afternoon.
- Take shifts on school or sports pick-ups and drop-offs for practices and games.
- Help with homework and school assignments.
- Listen to what's happening in their life.

44 **Support for aging parents**: if they are caregivers for their parents or other family members, remember to offer help out with their care.

45 **Caregivers relief**: if the person has a live-in partner, relative or friend taking care of them, remember to offer to relieve them for several hours, an evening, or a weekend so that they can have some personal time.

- Include their preferences in the meals you might bring or support you can provide.

Pets

Anyone who enjoys pets, knows that they require a lot of routine and specialized care. And an exercised, clean, healthy animal is a better companions than one who is out of sort because their needs aren't being met. If you enjoy pets, remember to offer to help with the following

46 **Pet exercise and play**: offer to walk a dog or play with their cat.

47 **Pet sitting**: take care of their pet for a weekend or another short period of time.

48 **Grooming**: find out what kind of routine grooming is needed and either do it yourself or take their pet to their groomer for them.

49 **Other pet services**: ask what special needs their animals have including, routine vet visits, delivering heavy bags of food or cat litter, or just having a new toy to help entertain their pet.

Seasonal Tasks

50 **Yard work:** All homeowners and many renters have yard work that needs to be done regularly based on the season. But also think about those special cleanup times such as fall yard preparation for winter or spring yard cleanup and mulching.

- Outdoor work is especially nice since it can be done without disturbing the individual or family.

51 **Seasonal decorations**: based on the way they are used to celebrating holidays, decorate a tree or hang decorative lights, create a yard display. Decorating the entranceway to their house or apartment to welcome them home from the hospital or rehab center may bring special joy. If you do decorate, remember to return and take down the decorations at the appropriate time.

52 **Special dates support**: dates like April 15 for taxes or mail-in voting for elections can be an extra burden for people with limited energy and health. It's quite possible they haven't even remembered these dates, or they are worrying about them and it's causing them great concern. Find out if they need help getting an extension or taking papers to an expert to complete.

Children Can Be a Supporter Too

Just like adults, many children have huge hearts and a desire to help others. It's important that when we're looking for ways to support people with cancer, that children be invited to contribute.

53 **Phone calls and especially video ones**: are a great way for a person to keep in touch with children they know and love. And most children of all ages love using them.

54 **Small, crafted gifts, painted pictures, handmade cards**: can brighten not only the face of a person with cancer, but also decorate the room where they spend a lot of time.

- I still keep a bright painted stone with the word "Hope" on it that magically appeared on my doorstep one morning. I still don't know who gifted this to me, but it warmed my heart when I received it and still makes me smile every time I walk past it.

Gifts

We all enjoy bringing someone a gift that will be appreciated and used. Here are special ideas for people with cancer.

55 **Medical appointment visits bag**: to take to their medical appointments and treatments. Fill it with a small soft blanket (size of airplane ones), water/juice, snack bars, simple reading material, sanitizer lotion, notebook/pen to write down doctor's notes or their own questions to ask a doctor.

- I can't tell you how often I sat for long periods of time in a reception room waiting to see a doctor or have another medical test or procedure performed. After being unprepared and uncomfortable for too many, I finally assembled my own medical visit bag. Its contents rescued me so many times.

- Many waiting and examination rooms feel cold to someone with a compromised body. My small blanket in my bag not only kept me warmer, but its softness and familiarity was soothing.
- I learned to take to each doctor visit my own list of questions or things I wanted to discuss. I not only used this list during my visit, but I also recorded the answers I received on a tablet I kept in my visit bag. It was helpful after a visit to read these notes again and use it for a reference when others asked me questions.

56 **Entertainment subscriptions based on their interests:** buy this kind of entertainment to fill long days of inactivity including TV or movie services, magazines, or audio books. Or offer to pick out and return books from the library if they have the energy to read.

57 **Home cleaning or yard service paid in advance**: this is an ideal group gift to keep a home functional.

58 **An in-home manicure/pedicure or haircut/styling**: providing or securing this kind of service to be done in their home is a wonderful way to make the person feel cared for and presentable.

59 **Gift cards of all kinds:** food delivery service, transportation, house cleaning, yard work, pet walking or grooming.

- Another great gift for people who want to support but don't have a lot of time.
- Also a great idea for non-local people.

60 **Self printed photos of them doing things they enjoy and with their loved ones:** is a great gift to take to them in a hospital or other medial/personal care facility.

- Download photos and print them on a home printer is a great way to share memories.
- Tape these to their bedside table or bed. Even home-printed photos can provide good memories and conversation starters for all who come into their room.
- Photos also give medical staff a view of the person when they were healthy, and a chance to reminisce for those that know them. Most importantly, these photos can be tossed when it's time to leave and return home, and it is more sanitary this way.

61 **Handmade comfort shawl or blanket:** can bring great warmth and comfort.

- My aunt who is a prolific crocheter sent me a comfort shawl she had crocheted herself. She had taken it to her church prayer group, and they had said prayers for healing while holding it.

- A shawl is an ideal gift for a person who wants to sit upright in bed or in a chair with a covering over their upper body.
- My shoulders always get cold. A shawl is perfect to keep shoulders warm and allow the user to still use their hands above their blankets.

As you read through these ideas, others likely came to mind. Simply think about your own weekly, monthly, and seasonal routines — then find ways to adapt them to make a real difference in the life of someone with cancer.

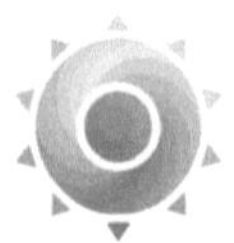

Timing of Assistance Offers

AT THE ONSET OF BEING DIAGNOSED with cancer or the beginning of a treatment like radiation or chemotherapy, word will get out as people learn about the person's medical challenges. And, offers will pour in from people who want to make the person's life with cancer easier.

On the receiving end of all these early offers, I was still busy processing what was happening and, thankfully, had no idea about the specific details or difficulties of the road ahead. I was incapable of accepting most offers or visualizing the kinds of assistance I'd need, as the treatments and/or cancer progressed. Mostly I just smiled, nodded my head acknowledging any offer, mumbled thanks, or said something like, "I'll let you know."

More importantly, later I couldn't remember who had offered what as I hadn't made a list of their names and types of offers.

About 50 years ago, after a huge flood when the Susquehanna River rose 38 feet and devastated miles of homes in Wilkes Barre, Pennsylvania, I volunteered to process applications for financial assistance for those affected by the flood.

Daily, long strings of buses arrived filled with clothing donated by well-meaning people in cities all over the United States. A large local high school gymnasium became filled with the voluminous donations. We had so much clothing that eventually city officials put out the message—no more buses or clothing donations. Thank you but we have plenty for now.

What was even more surprising—when people who had lost everything came to the school to get clothing for their family, most only picked out a single outfit for each child and themselves. We volunteers were surprised because it was obvious they were going to need a lot more clothing than one outfit, and the mounds of free clothing for taking without limitations were there in front of them.

But people were overwhelmed by their losses, in shock, and couldn't see beyond the current moment to the frightening future where many would have to start all over. For them, visualizing on-going needs wasn't possible.

At the beginning of my husband's diagnosis of only several months to live, I couldn't think about the resources I would soon need. I didn't want to imagine what the future would look like. But over time, as we found ways to extend his life to 11 months, a great variety of help would come to be appreciated.

At nine months the outside of our home clearly showed signs of neglect. When a friend called and said she and her husband were coming over on Saturday to do our fall gardening, I cried with relief and happiness. When they arrived, she quickly reviewed what they were prepared to do and asked for my approval. They even brought their own yard tools and trash bags. When they left, I needed to do nothing to clean up after them. And I had a beautiful front yard that no longer showed neglect.

An important point about supporting others—don't offer once, move on, and wait for a request. The longer the period the person is facing difficult therapies and the greater their health is impacted, the more they can use assistance.

During my first two cancers, I was able to navigate both surgeries easily. I even went to a neighborhood party two days after the first one. But six weeks post-surgery I began radiation five days a week for three weeks.

I chose to drive myself 45 miles in each direction to all 15 sessions, which meant driving on the crowded beltways around both Washington D.C. and then Baltimore, MD. The primary reason I chose to drive myself to all treatments is because I didn't want to entertain my volunteer driver with conversation or listen to the radio or music. I just needed silence.

Now, 13 years later, I realize how much work I needed to do on myself about being willing to accept help from others. If I had stated that I wanted drivers who could go without conversation and music (and we all know which people would be able to follow that kind of request), I wouldn't have needed to drive myself and risk a possible accident due to exhaustion.

Not everyone knows how to receive assistance. Be patient as you make your offers. The more sensitive you are to the person's needs, listening to what their energy is saying, and eliminating your need for gestures of appreciation, the more likely your offers will be welcomed.

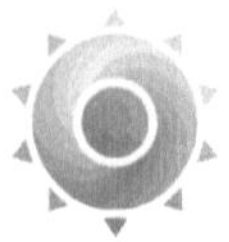

Caregivers— The Often Forgotten Ones

THIS SECTION WOULD not be complete without talking about caregivers and their personal needs for support. Many of the things that you do to support persons with cancer also help make their caregivers' lives easier. Often, caregivers feel they must put themselves second as they support the person with cancer. But they need their own separate support network to share their own experiences and feelings.

Recently my neighbor, who supported me through my chemo treatment with dozens of small gestures, unexpectedly had a husband in the hospital for several weeks, followed by another month at a care facility where he continued medical treatments and received physical therapy. This neighbor had local family and friends, so I knew that some support was already in place.

Every time I saw her though I'd say, "I want to know how your husband is doing, but first talk to me about yourself. How are you?" I'd then spend time listening to how she was coping, feeling, sleeping, eating, and how life in general was for her. Like many caregivers, she was glad to have time to think about herself and talk to a friend.

And as I listened, I noted what kinds of things I could do to make her life a bit easier.

As a caregiver for my husband during his cancer, I often found myself still in my pajamas in the middle of the afternoon. I hadn't had time to shower, get dressed, or even make something for myself to eat.

A primary need for many caregivers is simply to have a chance for a break from the person they are caring for. Even as short a period of time as an hour can be helpful.

One caregiver friend wished for time to go out on one of his former daily runs. Another needed time to do errands. Having someone the caregiver trusts who can stay with their loved one while they take time for themselves is a much needed gift.

And if two people want to join in helping a caregiver, why not arrange for one to take the caregiver to lunch, shopping, movie, or a walk while the other stays with the person with cancer?

FINAL WORDS

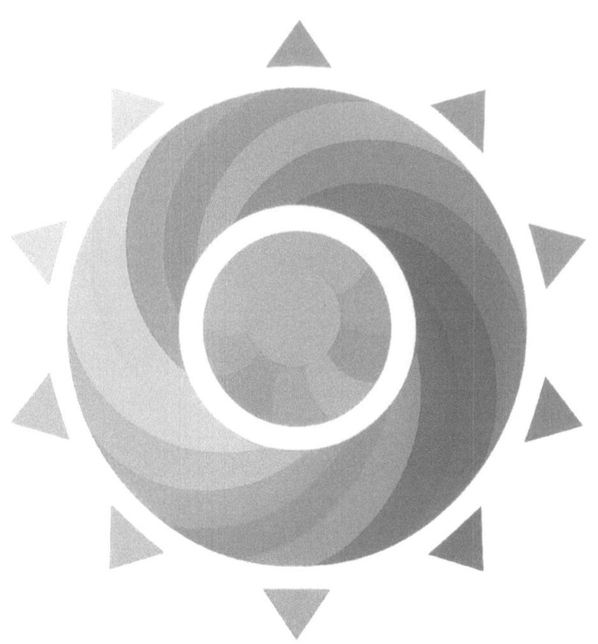

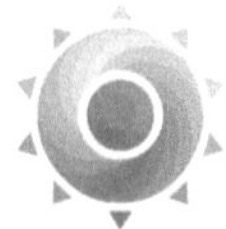

Assisting Others

WE ALL WANT TO MAKE the cancer journey easier for others, especially for those we know and care about.

But the goal of communicating with people with cancer and supporting them shouldn't be to make a significant difference in a person's life through one magnanimous gesture. We all enjoy receiving immediate feedback that what we've said or done is perfect. But that isn't why we're offering our help.

Instead, your biggest contributions may be by performing a series of much smaller actions over time that help in little ways.

Also, just by continuing to interact and talk with a person who has cancer about normal things you've shared or enjoyed in the past, you will help keep that relationship current. And you will assist them in not feeling alone or disconnected from their former life.

Some people with cancer will never be finished with it. Some will continue to need cancer therapies for the rest of their lives, or until new solutions for their kind of cancer are found and available.

A too-often expressed statement by some people with cancer is, "I've exhausted all of my offers for help, but I still have some of the same support needs as when I was first diagnosed."

For long-time caregivers and dedicated volunteers, experiencing "supporter fatigue" is common when support continues for years. Don't assume that a person has enough help when their cancer journey continues for longer periods of time. Their current supporters may need a break, or the numbers of earlier supporters may have slowly dwindled.

If you are able and willing, don't just respond with offers of help solely to newly diagnosed persons with cancer. Check in again with people you've helped in the past to see what types of support they need now.

Unfortunately, it not only takes a community to raise children, but it also takes dedicated supporters to aid people with long-term cancer.

There are so many medical advances in cancer happening daily. The focus on ending cancer that began in the 1970s has continued, and there is real progress being made. Unfortunately, also growing is the percentage of the population being diagnosed with cancer.

It's our collective wish that ways to identify, treat, and end cancer will no longer just be a dream or goal, but an actual reality.

All of us need to learn more about cancer so that fear isn't our initial and primary reaction when we hear about it.

When we use cancer etiquette as guidelines for what to say and not say, and when we volunteer to support people with cancer in a wide variety of ways, we can collectively make a difference in people with cancer's lives.

Hopefully, you now have even better and more effective ideas for how to make life easier for people with cancer.

Never forget—the person you are supporting is an amazing person who is more than just their disease.

About the Author

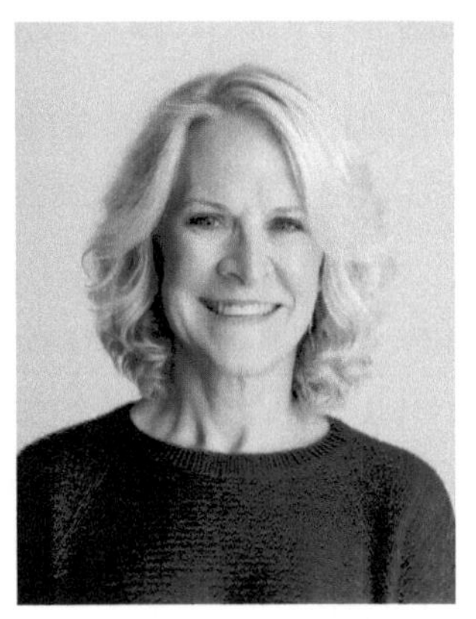

Linda Crill faced cancer three times and served as caregiver to her husband with terminal cancer, giving her an intimate understanding of both sides of the cancer experience. She has listened to countless stories in support groups and at large cancer gatherings, deepening her insight into the everyday challenges people with cancer face.

As a professional speaker and organizational development facilitator, she has helped Fortune 500 companies and associations navigate accelerating change and answer "What now?" when the unexpected presents itself.

Today she brings that expertise to the cancer community, speaking at conferences, cancer events, and retreats on the often-overlooked topic of how families, friends, and coworkers can better support people with cancer.

Her cancer insights have been featured on NBC, ABC, and Fox, published in national magazines and digital media, and shared in keynote presentations and workshops at major events, including serving as keynote speaker for *Breast Cancer Wellness* magazine's Thrivers Cruises.

www.LindaCrill.com

Also by Linda Crill

Blind Curves—One Woman's Unusual Journey to Reinvent Herself and Answer What Now?
A memoir about navigating loss, daring to take risks, and discovering new possibilities after life's unexpected turns.

Note: Also republished in 2014 by Skyhorse Publishing under the subtitle: *A Woman, a Motorcycle, and a Journey to Reinvent Herself.*

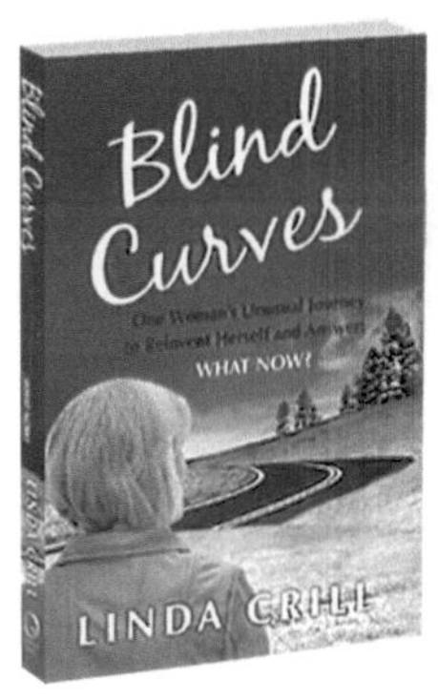

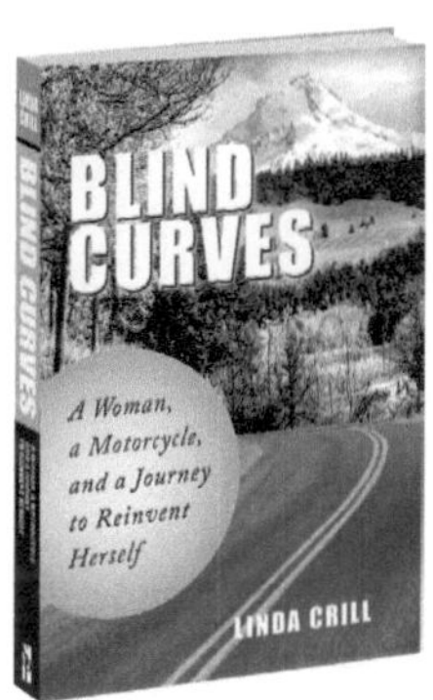

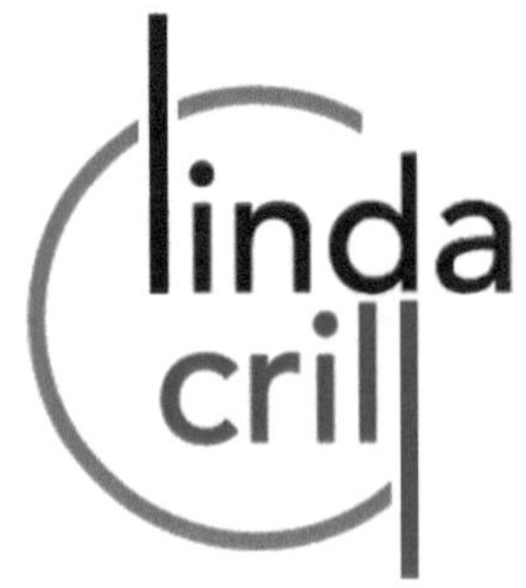

Stay Connected

Thank you for reading *Cancer InsideOut*. I'd love to continue the conversation.

For resources, updates, speaking invitations, or to schedule an online book club discussion, please visit:

www.CancerInsideOut.com or simply scan the code below with your phone.

Scan code to visit CancerInsideOut.com

www.ingramcontent.com/pod-product-compliance
Ingram Content Group UK Ltd.
Pitfield, Milton Keynes, MK11 3LW, UK
UKHW040243300726
14061UKWH00002BD/131

9 780985 898540